okay! thinner thighs for everyone

More Sylvia by Nicole Hollander

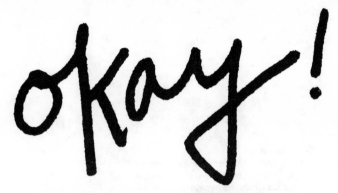

okay!

thinner thighs
for everyone

By Nicole Hollander

St. Martin's Press, New York

Book designed by
Tom Greensfelder and Dolores Wilber

ISBN 0-312-58316-8

First Edition
10 9 8 7 6 5 4 3 2 1

Nicole Hollander's greeting cards are available from
The Maine Line Co., P.O. Box 418, Rockport, ME 04856. (207) 236-8536.

OKAY. I KNOW YOU'RE GOING to FIND tHIS HARD to BELIEVE, BUT I'VE BEEN UP FOR HOURS. I WASHED tHE FLOOR, I WROTE 2 CHAPTERS OF MY NOVEL...

This book is dedicated to those who, for whatever reason, are still in their bathrobes when the mail carrier comes to call.

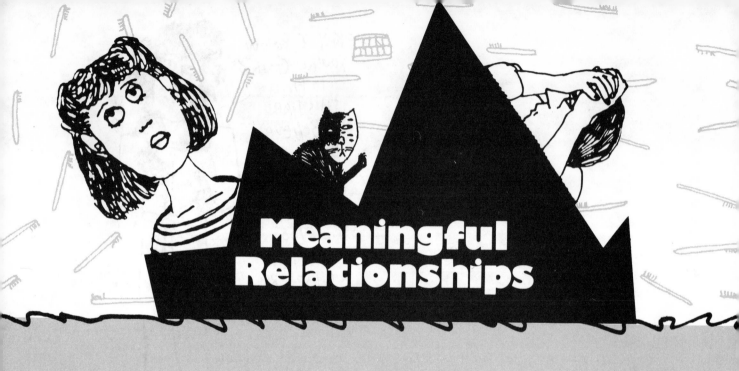

Meaningful Relationships

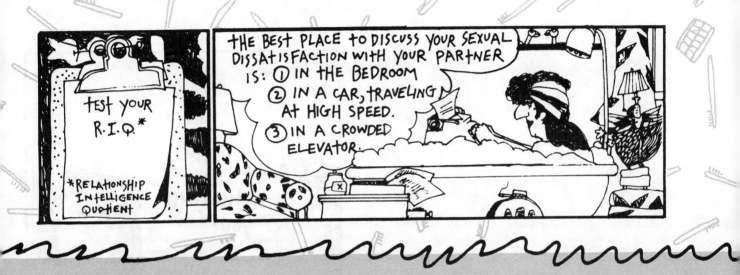

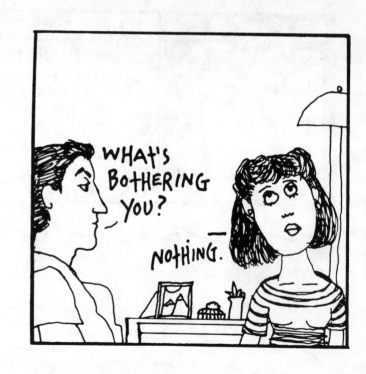

THERE IS SOMETHING WRONG; I CAN ALWAYS TELL. YOU'RE HOLDING IT IN. ITS JUST GOING TO GET WORSE AND WORSE. IT DRIVES ME CRAZY! TELL ME.

WHEN YOU WERE SHAVING THIS MORNING, I NOTICED YOU HAVE A TINY NORFOLK PINE TREE GROWING OUT OF THE SMALL OF YOUR BACK.

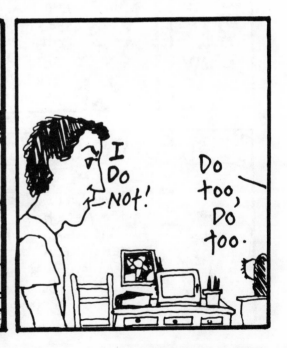

I DO NOT!

DO TOO, DO TOO.

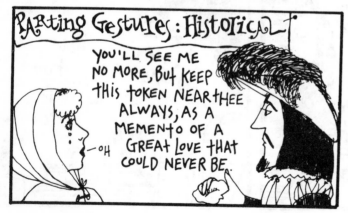

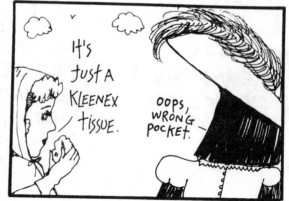

10

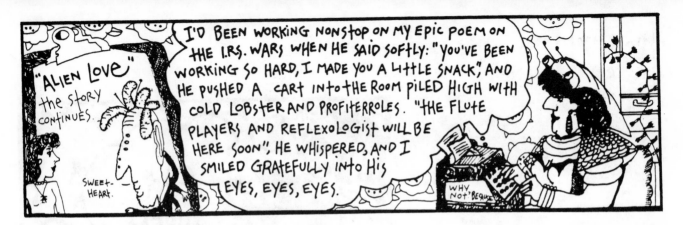

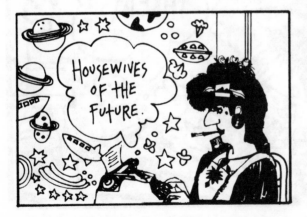

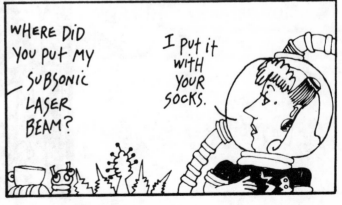

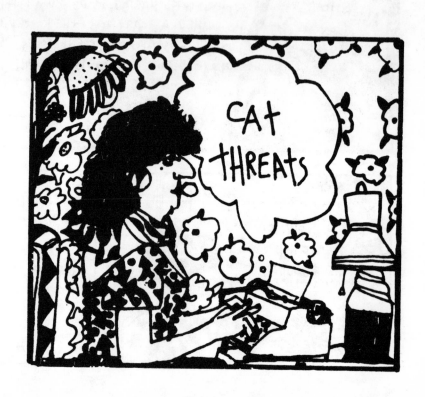

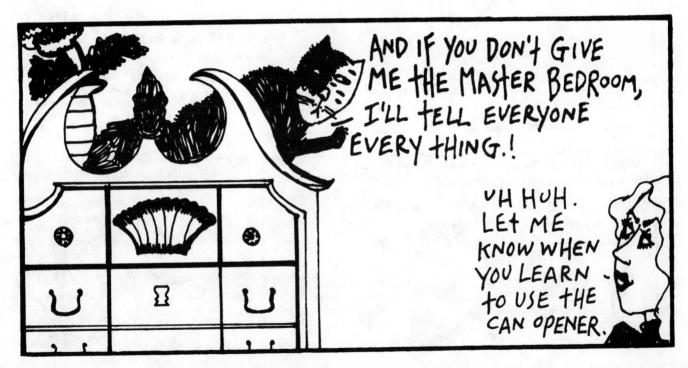

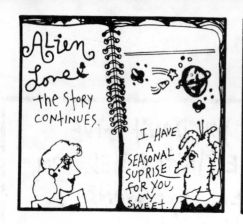

Alien Love: the story continues.

I HAVE A SEASONAL SUPRISE FOR YOU, MY SWEET.

"I KNOW YOU'RE HOMESICK FOR EARTH AND ESPECIALLY CHICAGO THIS TIME OF YEAR", HE MURMURED (PRONOUNCING IT "DRCHIVAGO" WITH THAT DELIGHTFUL LISP THAT THE MEN OF HIS PLANET HAVE). HE LED ME OUT TO THE PATIO AND FLICKED A SWITCH... SLOWLY AND BEAUTIFULLY IT BEGAN TO SNOW. "LATER SOME MEN WILL COME AND FIGHT OVER PARKING SPACES", HE SAID, KISSING MY EYELIDS.

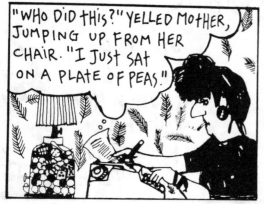

"WHO DID THIS?" YELLED MOTHER, JUMPING UP FROM HER CHAIR. "I JUST SAT ON A PLATE OF PEAS."

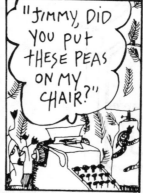

"JIMMY, DID YOU PUT THESE PEAS ON MY CHAIR?"

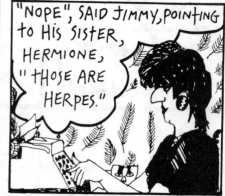

"NOPE", SAID JIMMY, POINTING TO HIS SISTER, HERMIONE, "THOSE ARE HERPES."

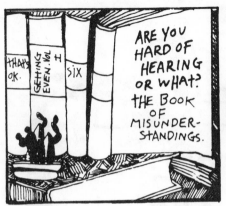

ARE YOU HARD OF HEARING OR WHAT? THE BOOK OF MISUNDERSTANDINGS.

(book spines: that's OK. GETTING EVEN VOL. H, SIX)

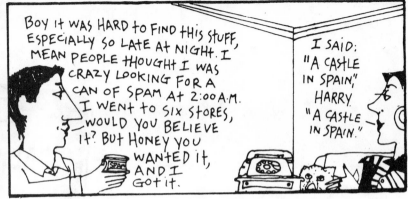

BOY IT WAS HARD TO FIND THIS STUFF, ESPECIALLY SO LATE AT NIGHT. I MEAN PEOPLE THOUGHT I WAS CRAZY LOOKING FOR A CAN OF SPAM AT 2:00 A.M. I WENT TO SIX STORES, WOULD YOU BELIEVE IT? BUT HONEY YOU WANTED IT, AND I GOT IT.

I SAID: "A CASTLE IN SPAIN," HARRY. "A CASTLE IN SPAIN."

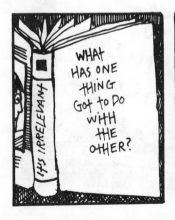

WHAT HAS ONE THING GOT TO DO WITH THE OTHER?

(book spine: IT'S IRRELEVANT)

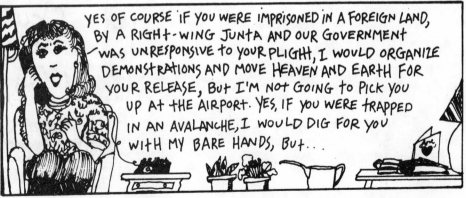

YES OF COURSE IF YOU WERE IMPRISONED IN A FOREIGN LAND, BY A RIGHT-WING JUNTA AND OUR GOVERNMENT WAS UNRESPONSIVE TO YOUR PLIGHT, I WOULD ORGANIZE DEMONSTRATIONS AND MOVE HEAVEN AND EARTH FOR YOUR RELEASE, BUT I'M NOT GOING TO PICK YOU UP AT THE AIRPORT. YES, IF YOU WERE TRAPPED IN AN AVALANCHE, I WOULD DIG FOR YOU WITH MY BARE HANDS, BUT...

15

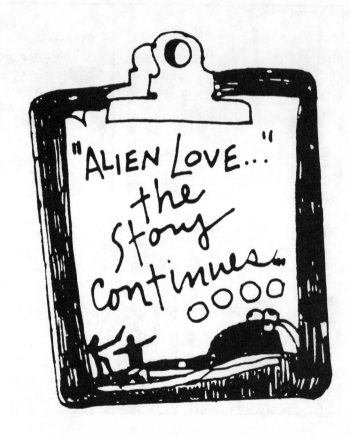

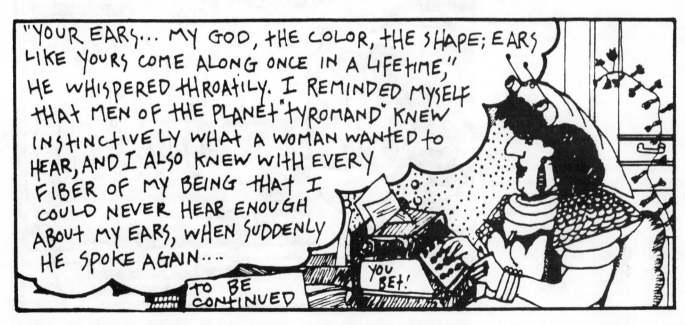

17

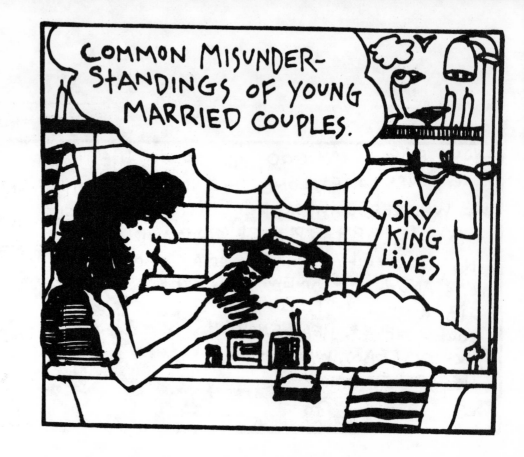

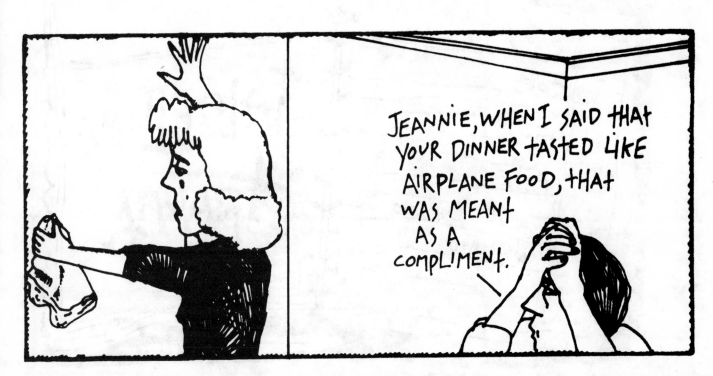

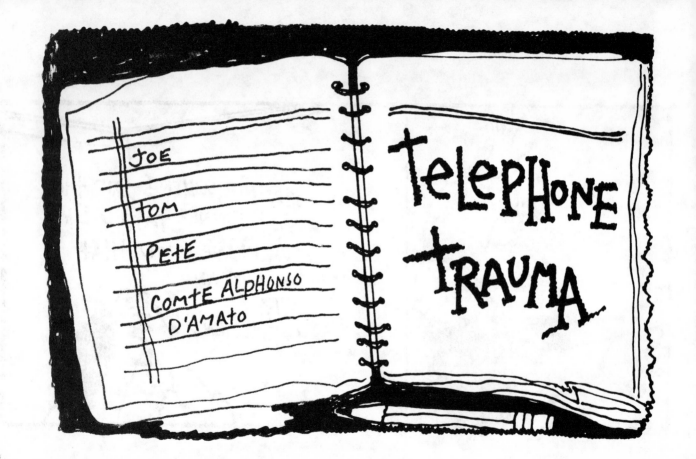

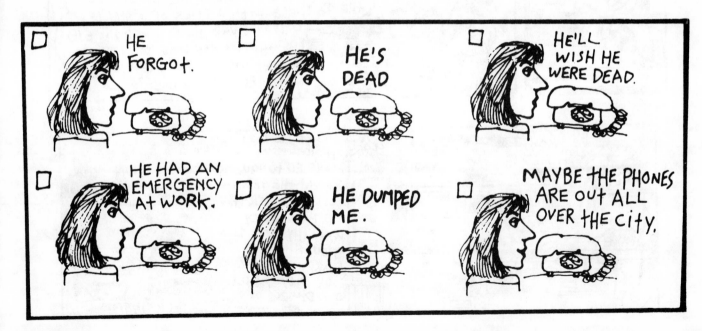

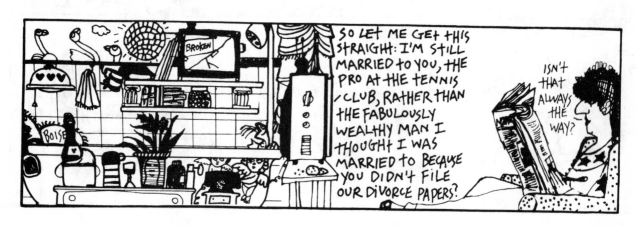
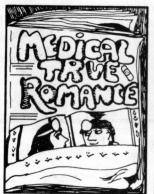
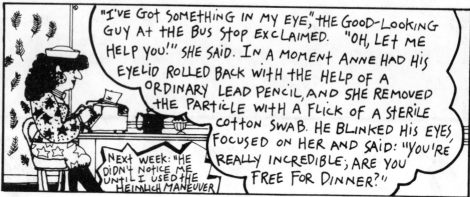

Alien Love
CHAPTER 5:
UNLOOKED FOR
EVENTS

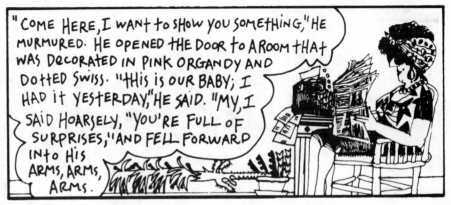

"COME HERE, I WANT to SHOW YOU SOMETHING," HE MURMURED. HE OPENED THE DOOR TO A ROOM THAT WAS DECORATED IN PINK ORGANDY AND DOTTED SWISS. "THIS IS OUR BABY; I HAD IT YESTERDAY," HE SAID. "MY, I SAID HOARSELY, "YOU'RE FULL OF SURPRISES," AND FELL FORWARD INTO HIS ARMS, ARMS, ARMS.

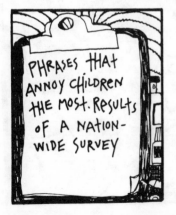

PHRASES THAT ANNOY CHILDREN THE MOST. RESULTS OF A NATION-WIDE SURVEY

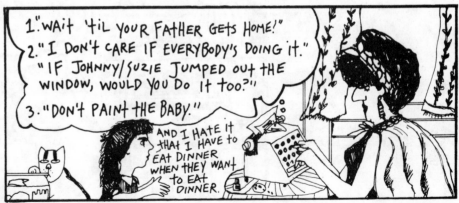

1. "WAIT 'TIL YOUR FATHER GETS HOME!"
2. "I DON'T CARE IF EVERYBODY'S DOING IT." "IF JOHNNY/SUZIE JUMPED OUT THE WINDOW, WOULD YOU DO IT TOO?"
3. "DON'T PAINT THE BABY."

AND I HATE IT THAT I HAVE TO EAT DINNER WHEN THEY WANT TO EAT DINNER.

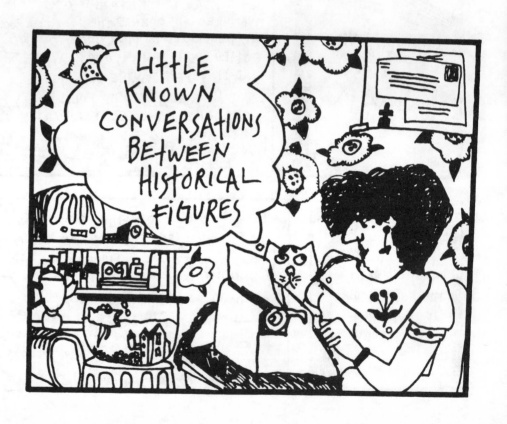

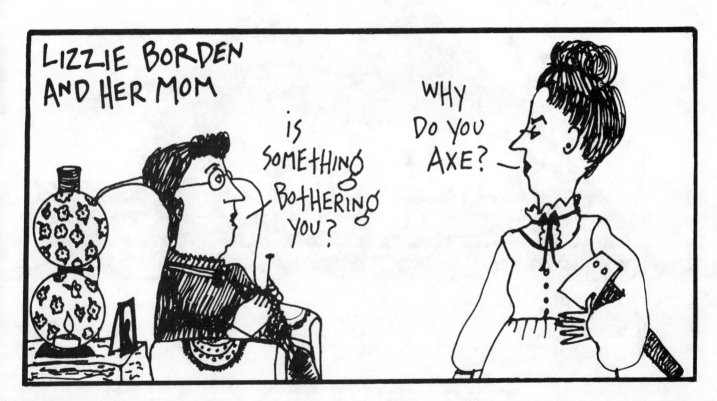

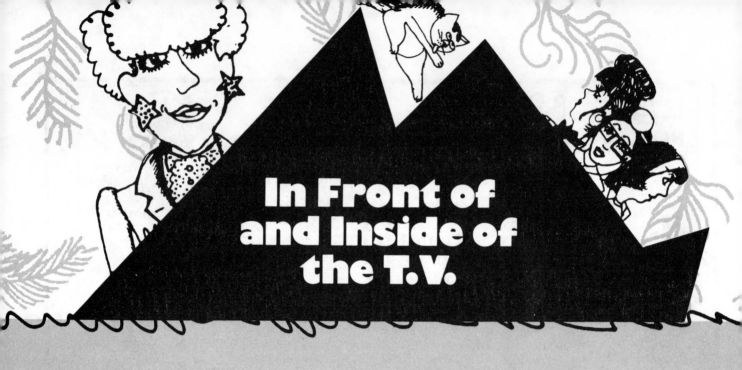

In Front of and Inside of the T.V.

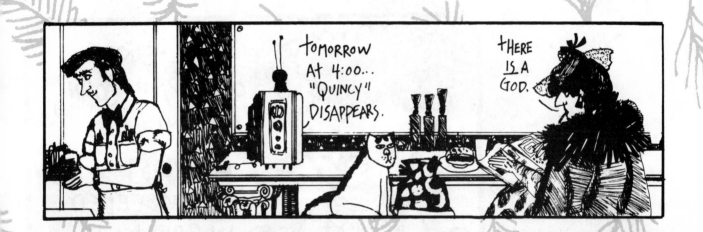

27

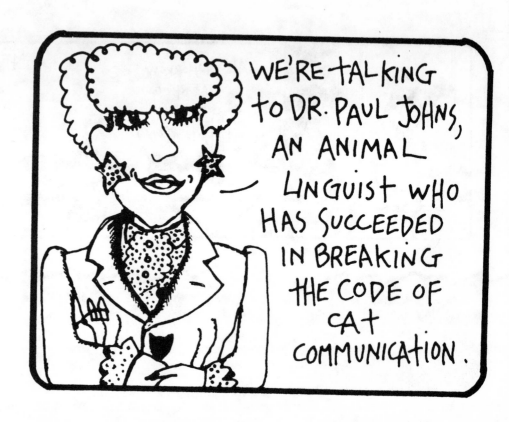

28

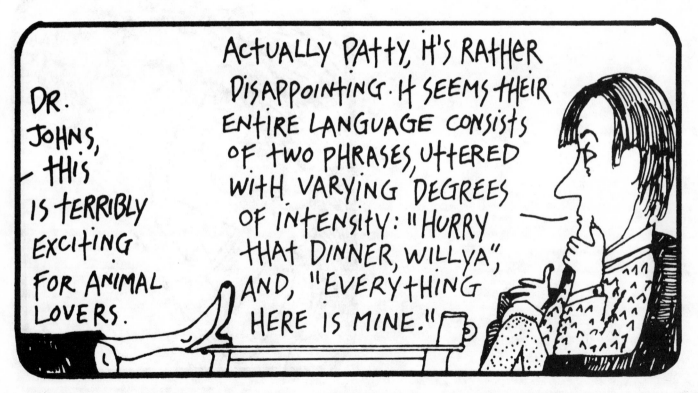

DR. JOHNS, THIS IS TERRIBLY EXCITING FOR ANIMAL LOVERS.

ACTUALLY PATTY, IT'S RATHER DISAPPOINTING. IT SEEMS THEIR ENTIRE LANGUAGE CONSISTS OF TWO PHRASES, UTTERED WITH VARYING DEGREES OF INTENSITY: "HURRY THAT DINNER, WILLYA", AND, "EVERYTHING HERE IS MINE."

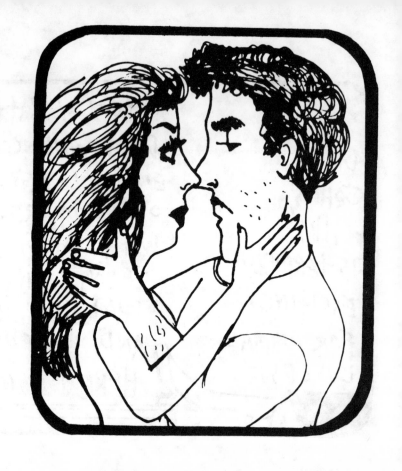

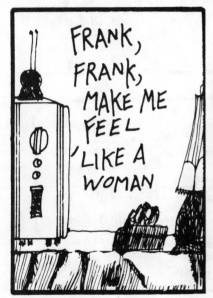
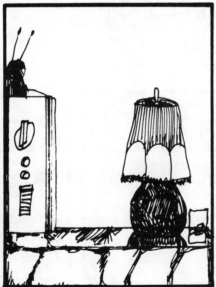
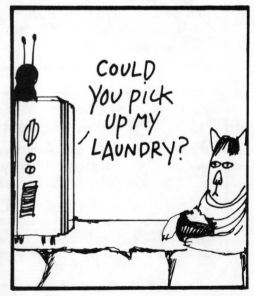

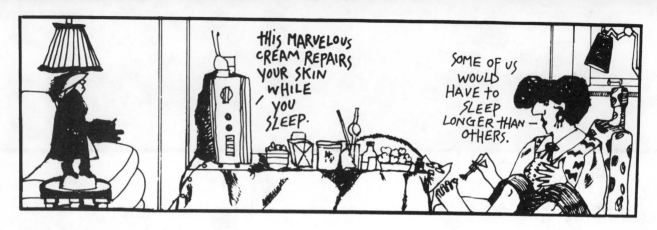

THIS MARVELOUS CREAM REPAIRS YOUR SKIN WHILE YOU SLEEP.

SOME OF US WOULD HAVE TO SLEEP LONGER THAN — OTHERS.

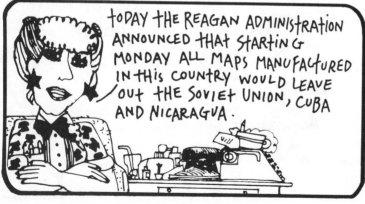

TODAY THE REAGAN ADMINISTRATION ANNOUNCED THAT STARTING MONDAY ALL MAPS MANUFACTURED IN THIS COUNTRY WOULD LEAVE OUT THE SOVIET UNION, CUBA AND NICARAGUA.

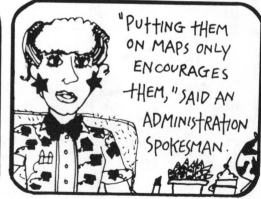

"PUTTING THEM ON MAPS ONLY ENCOURAGES THEM," SAID AN ADMINISTRATION SPOKESMAN.

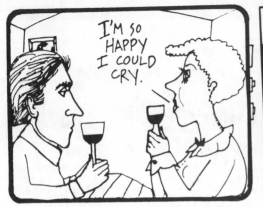

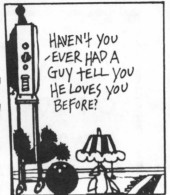

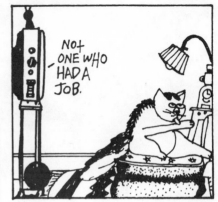

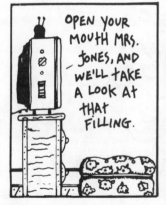

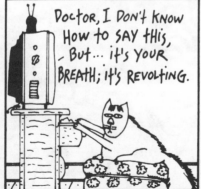

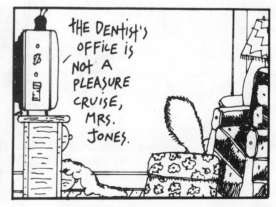

Lives of Susan

COMEDY MINI-SERIES ABOUT A WOMAN WHO HAS A 3-WAY SPLIT PERSONALITY: COCKTAIL WAITRESS, HOUSEWIFE AND CHIROPRACTOR.

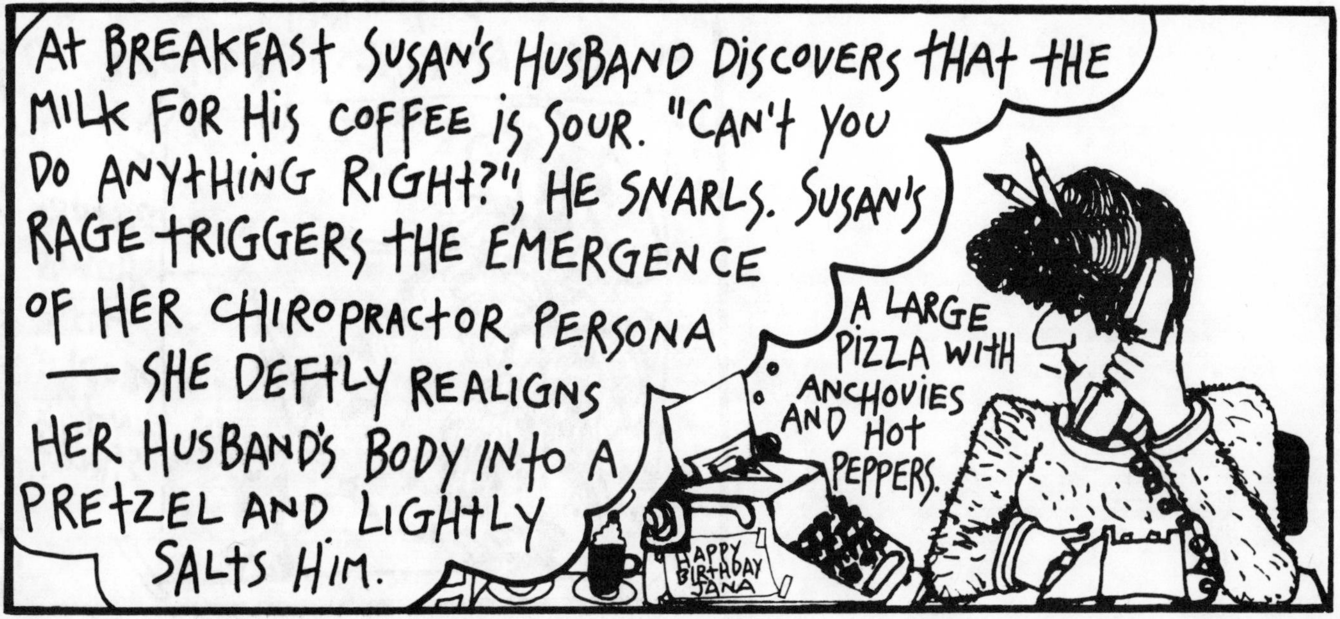
AT BREAKFAST SUSAN'S HUSBAND DISCOVERS THAT THE MILK FOR HIS COFFEE IS SOUR. "CAN'T YOU DO ANYTHING RIGHT?", HE SNARLS. SUSAN'S RAGE TRIGGERS THE EMERGENCE OF HER CHIROPRACTOR PERSONA — SHE DEFTLY REALIGNS HER HUSBAND'S BODY INTO A PRETZEL AND LIGHTLY SALTS HIM.
A LARGE PIZZA WITH ANCHOVIES AND HOT PEPPERS.
HAPPY BIRTHDAY JANA

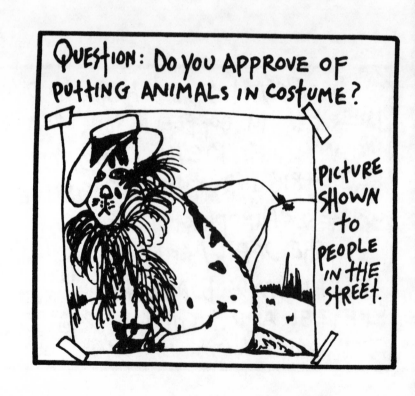

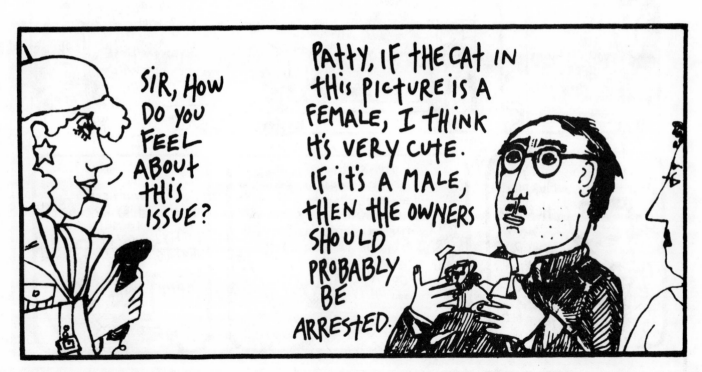

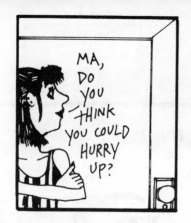

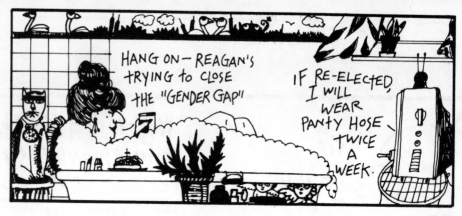

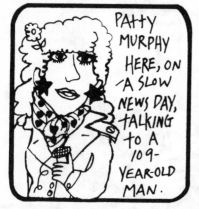

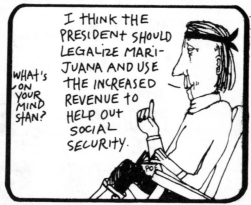

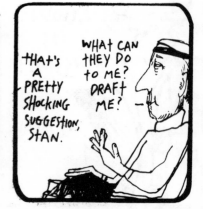

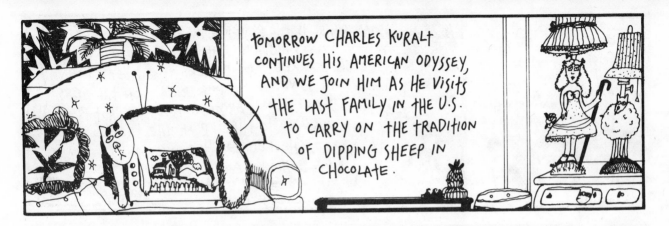

TOMORROW CHARLES KURALT CONTINUES HIS AMERICAN ODYSSEY, AND WE JOIN HIM AS HE VISITS THE LAST FAMILY IN THE U.S. TO CARRY ON THE TRADITION OF DIPPING SHEEP IN CHOCOLATE.

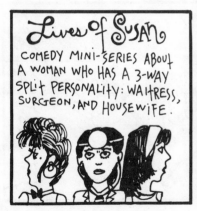

Lives of Susan

COMEDY MINI-SERIES ABOUT A WOMAN WHO HAS A 3-WAY SPLIT PERSONALITY: WAITRESS, SURGEON, AND HOUSEWIFE.

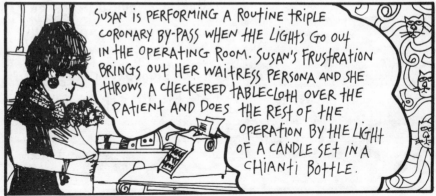

SUSAN IS PERFORMING A ROUTINE TRIPLE CORONARY BY-PASS WHEN THE LIGHTS GO OUT IN THE OPERATING ROOM. SUSAN'S FRUSTRATION BRINGS OUT HER WAITRESS PERSONA AND SHE THROWS A CHECKERED TABLECLOTH OVER THE PATIENT AND DOES THE REST OF THE OPERATION BY THE LIGHT OF A CANDLE SET IN A CHIANTI BOTTLE.

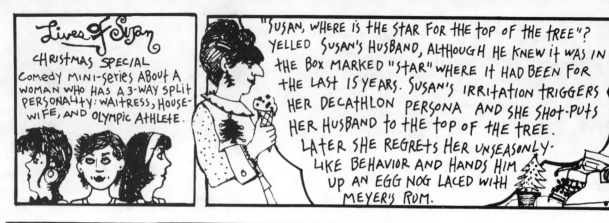

Lives of Susan

CHRISTMAS SPECIAL
Comedy mini-series about a woman who has a 3-way split personality: waitress, housewife, and Olympic athlete.

"Susan, where is the star for the top of the tree"? yelled Susan's husband, although he knew it was in the box marked "star" where it had been for the last 15 years. Susan's irritation triggers her decathlon persona and she shot-puts her husband to the top of the tree. Later she regrets her unseasonly-like behavior and hands him up an egg nog laced with Meyer's Rum.

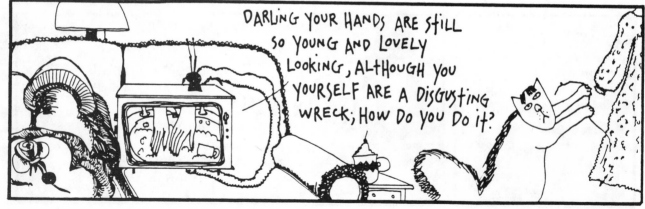

Darling your hands are still so young and lovely looking, although you yourself are a disgusting wreck; how do you do it?

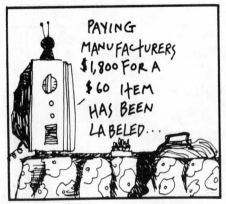

PAYING MANUFACTURERS $1,800 FOR A $60 ITEM HAS BEEN LABELED...

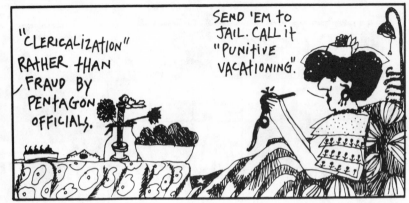

"CLERICALIZATION" RATHER THAN FRAUD BY PENTAGON OFFICIALS.

SEND 'EM TO JAIL. CALL IT "PUNITIVE VACATIONING".

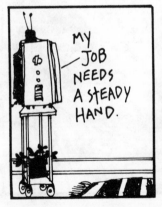

MY JOB NEEDS A STEADY HAND.

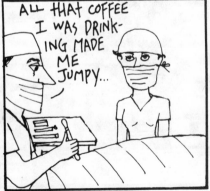

ALL THAT COFFEE I WAS DRINKING MADE ME JUMPY...

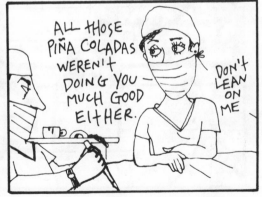

ALL THOSE PIÑA COLADAS WEREN'T DOING YOU MUCH GOOD EITHER.

DON'T LEAN ON ME

41

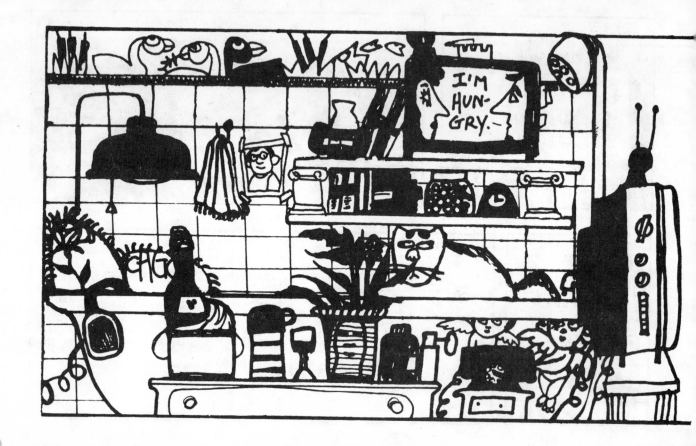

42

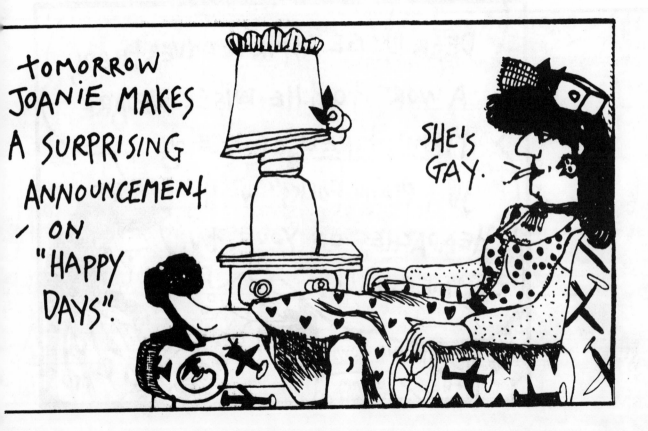

43

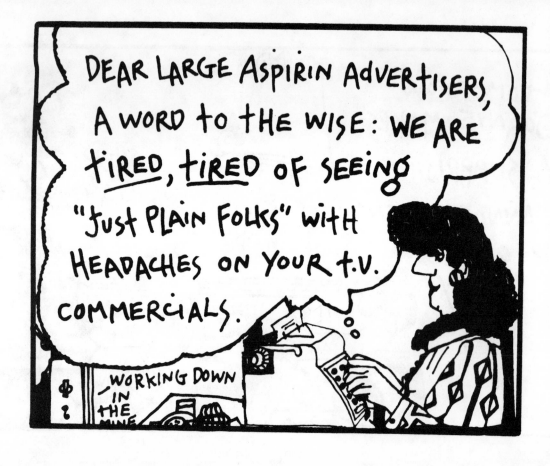

44

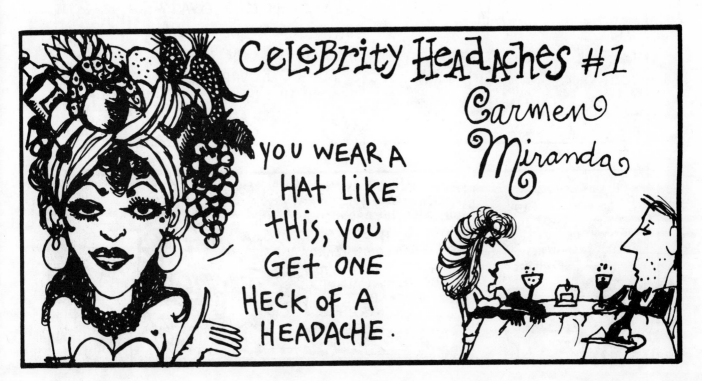

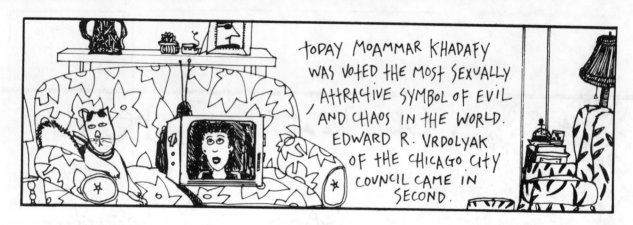

TODAY MOAMMAR KHADAFY WAS VOTED THE MOST SEXUALLY ATTRACTIVE SYMBOL OF EVIL AND CHAOS IN THE WORLD. EDWARD R. VRDOLYAK OF THE CHICAGO CITY COUNCIL CAME IN SECOND.

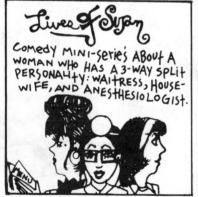

Lives of Susan

COMEDY MINI-SERIES ABOUT A WOMAN WHO HAS A 3-WAY SPLIT PERSONALITY: WAITRESS, HOUSEWIFE, AND ANESTHESIOLOGIST.

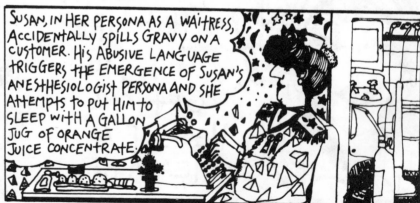

SUSAN, IN HER PERSONA AS A WAITRESS, ACCIDENTALLY SPILLS GRAVY ON A CUSTOMER. HIS ABUSIVE LANGUAGE TRIGGERS THE EMERGENCE OF SUSAN'S ANESTHESIOLOGIST PERSONA AND SHE ATTEMPTS TO PUT HIM TO SLEEP WITH A GALLON JUG OF ORANGE JUICE CONCENTRATE.

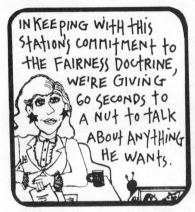 IN KEEPING WITH THIS STATION'S COMMITMENT TO THE FAIRNESS DOCTRINE, WE'RE GIVING 60 SECONDS TO A NUT TO TALK ABOUT ANYTHING HE WANTS.

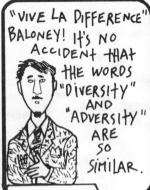 "VIVE LA DIFFERENCE" BALONEY! IT'S NO ACCIDENT THAT THE WORDS "DIVERSITY" AND "ADVERSITY" ARE SO SIMILAR.

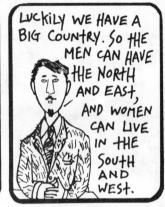 LUCKILY WE HAVE A BIG COUNTRY. SO THE MEN CAN HAVE THE NORTH AND EAST, AND WOMEN CAN LIVE IN THE SOUTH AND WEST.

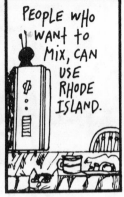 PEOPLE WHO WANT TO MIX, CAN USE RHODE ISLAND.

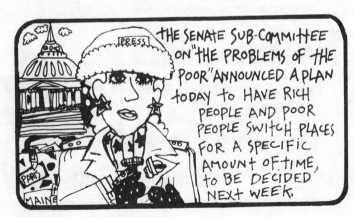 PRESS

THE SENATE SUB-COMMITTEE ON "THE PROBLEMS OF THE POOR" ANNOUNCED A PLAN TODAY TO HAVE RICH PEOPLE AND POOR PEOPLE SWITCH PLACES FOR A SPECIFIC AMOUNT OF TIME, TO BE DECIDED NEXT WEEK.

PARIS

MAINE

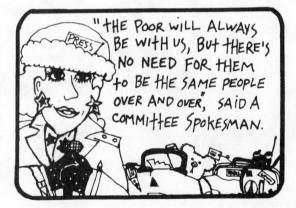 PRESS

"THE POOR WILL ALWAYS BE WITH US, BUT THERE'S NO NEED FOR THEM TO BE THE SAME PEOPLE OVER AND OVER", SAID A COMMITTEE SPOKESMAN.

47

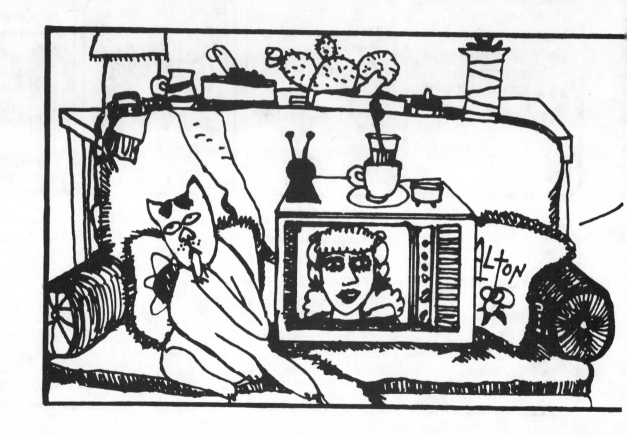

48

TODAY PRESIDENT REAGAN ANGRILY ANNOUNCED THAT IF THE CHINESE GOVERNMENT PROHIBITS THEIR PEOPLE FROM DRINKING COCA COLA, AMERICANS WOULD STOP BUYING ANY DRINKS THAT CAME WITH TINY PAPER UMBRELLAS IN THEM.

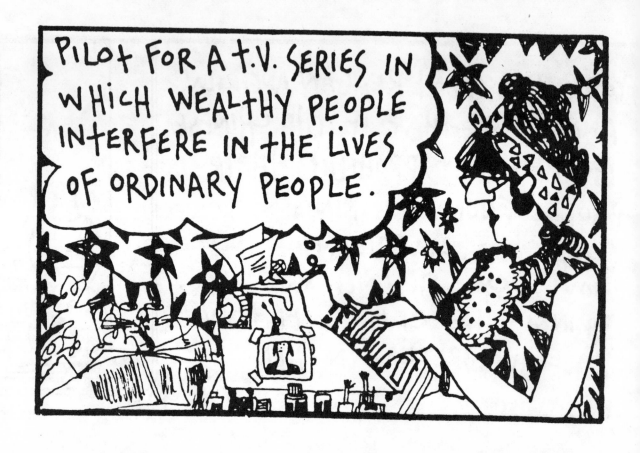

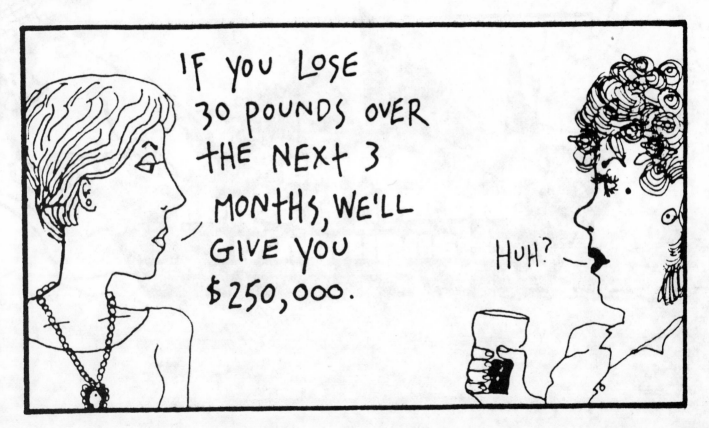

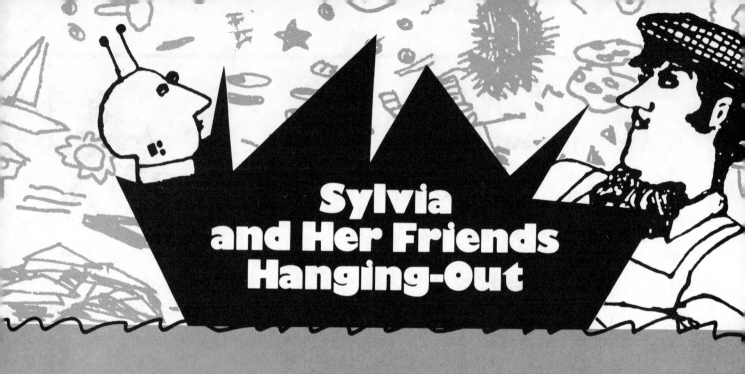

Sylvia and Her Friends Hanging-Out

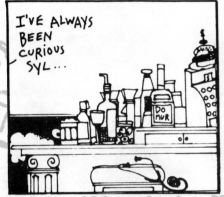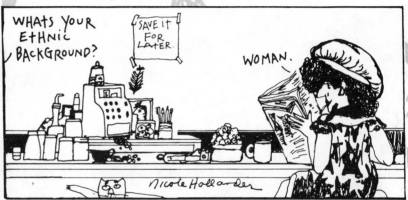

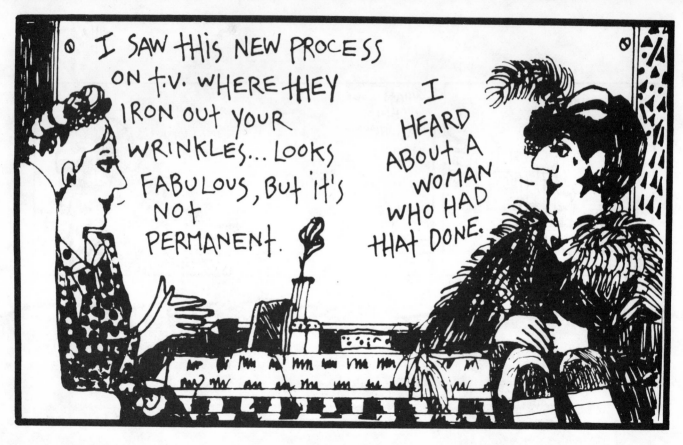

54

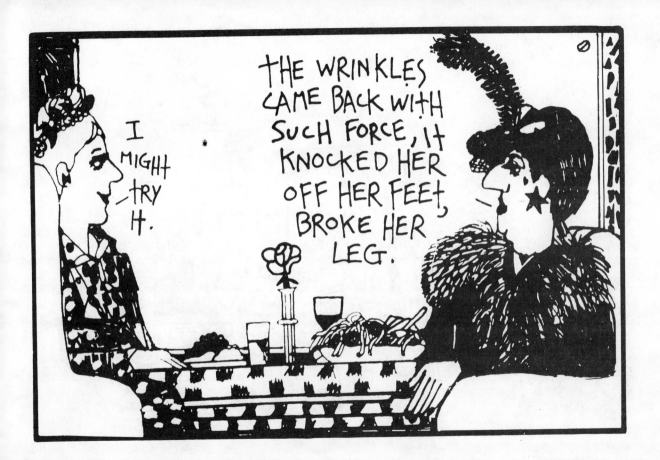

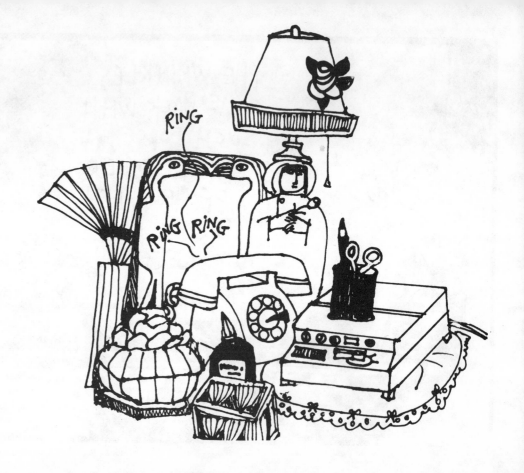

56

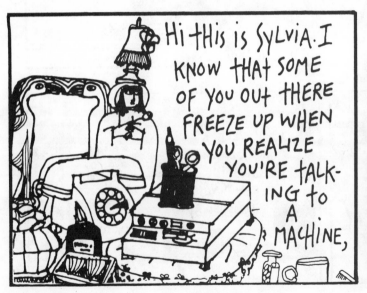
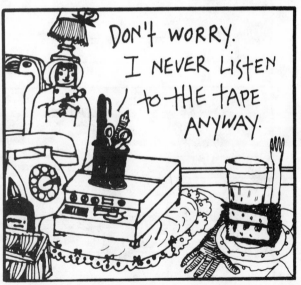

57

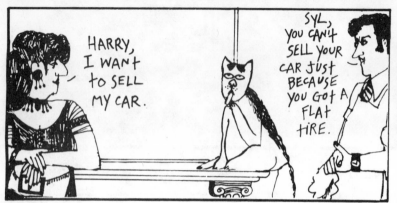

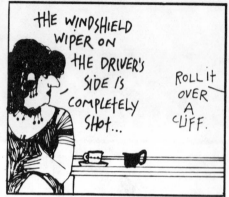

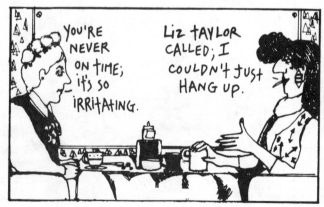

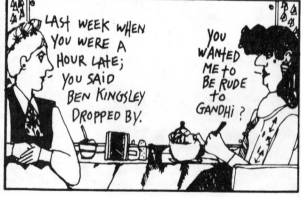

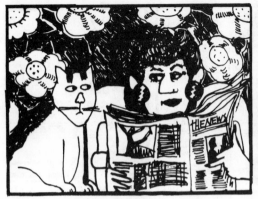
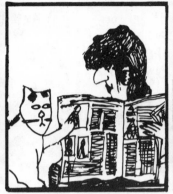
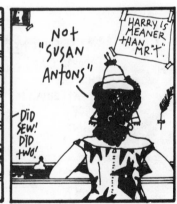

I DON'T WANT TO DO MY PETER LORRE IMITATION NOW.

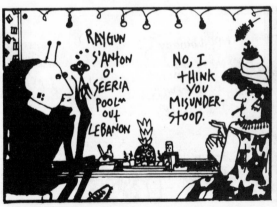

RAYGUN S'ANTON O' SEERIA POOL™ OUT LEBANON

NO, I THINK YOU MISUNDERSTOOD.

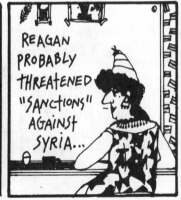

REAGAN PROBABLY THREATENED "SANCTIONS" AGAINST SYRIA...

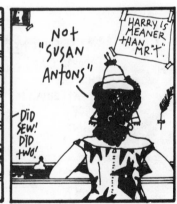

NOT "SUSAN ANTONS"

DID SEW! DID TWO!

HARRY IS MEANER THAN MR. T.

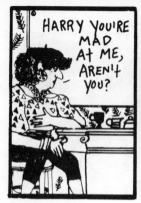

HARRY YOU'RE MAD AT ME, AREN'T YOU?

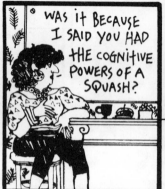

WAS IT BECAUSE I SAID YOU HAD THE COGNITIVE POWERS OF A SQUASH?

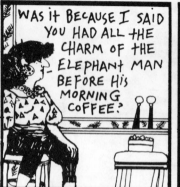

WAS IT BECAUSE I SAID YOU HAD ALL THE CHARM OF THE ELEPHANT MAN BEFORE HIS MORNING COFFEE?

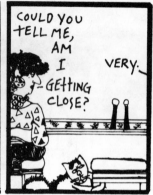

COULD YOU TELL ME, AM I GETTING CLOSE?

VERY.

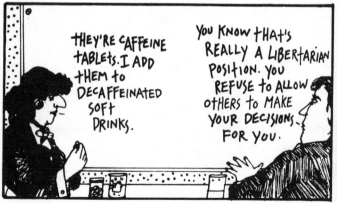

THEY'RE CAFFEINE TABLETS. I ADD THEM TO DECAFFEINATED SOFT DRINKS.

YOU KNOW THAT'S REALLY A LIBERTARIAN POSITION. YOU REFUSE TO ALLOW OTHERS TO MAKE YOUR DECISIONS FOR YOU.

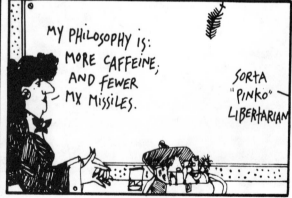

MY PHILOSOPHY IS: MORE CAFFEINE; AND FEWER MX MISSILES.

SORTA "PINKO" LIBERTARIAN

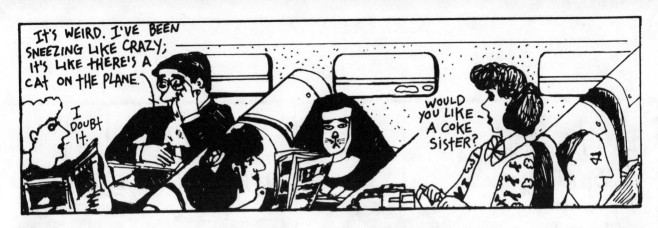

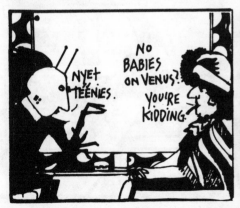

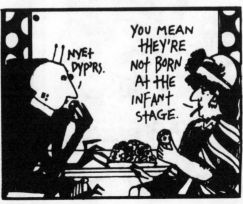

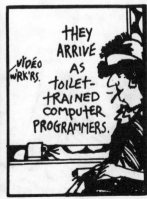

61

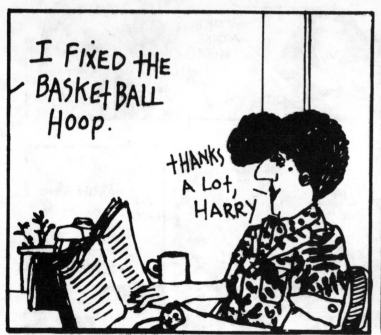

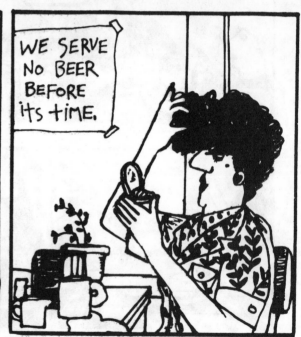

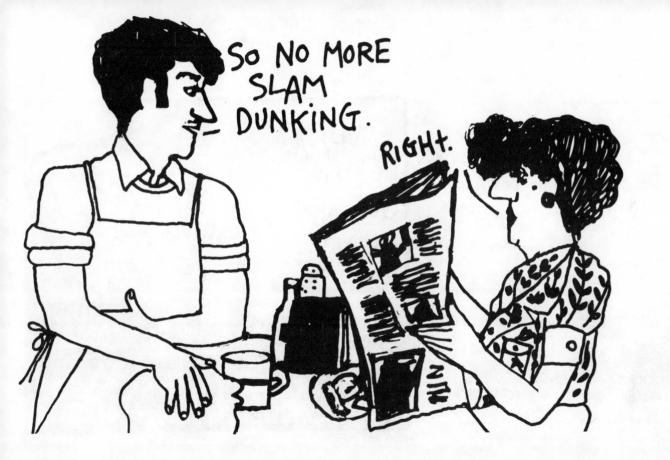

63

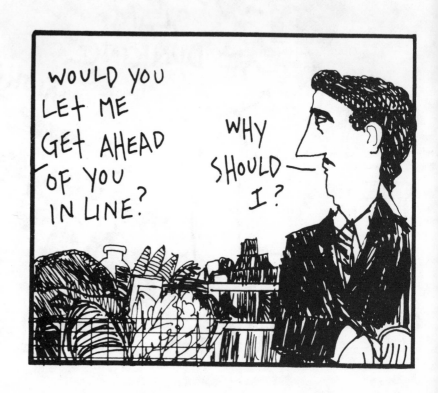

64

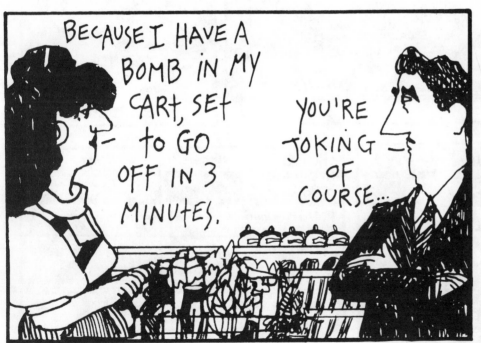
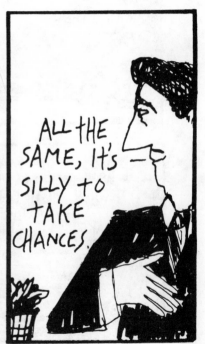

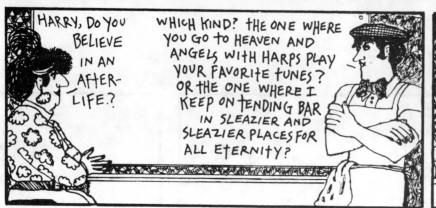

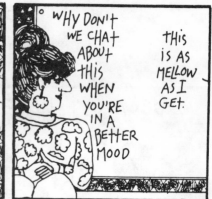

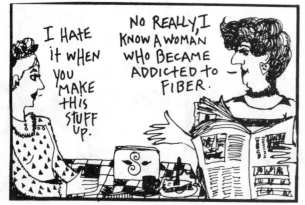

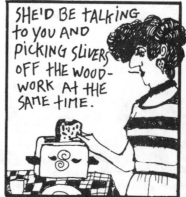

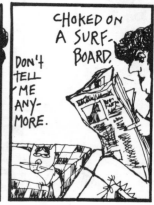

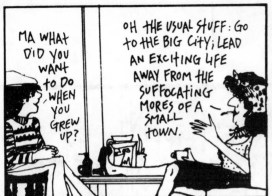

MA WHAT DID YOU WANT TO DO WHEN YOU GREW UP?

OH THE USUAL STUFF: GO TO THE BIG CITY; LEAD AN EXCITING LIFE AWAY FROM THE SUFFOCATING MORES OF A SMALL TOWN.

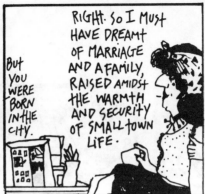

BUT YOU WERE BORN IN THE CITY.

RIGHT. SO I MUST HAVE DREAMT OF MARRIAGE AND A FAMILY, RAISED AMIDST THE WARMTH AND SECURITY OF SMALL TOWN LIFE.

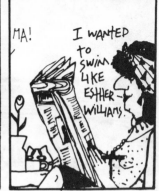

MA!

I WANTED TO SWIM LIKE ESTHER WILLIAMS.

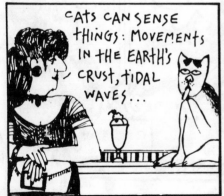

CATS CAN SENSE THINGS: MOVEMENTS IN THE EARTH'S CRUST, TIDAL WAVES...

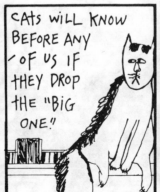

CATS WILL KNOW BEFORE ANY OF US IF THEY DROP THE "BIG ONE!"

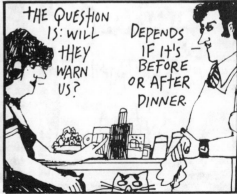

THE QUESTION IS: WILL THEY WARN US?

DEPENDS IF IT'S BEFORE OR AFTER DINNER.

67

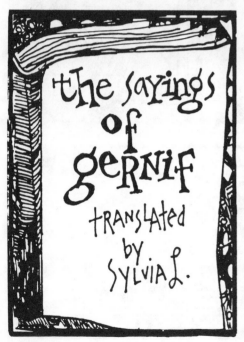

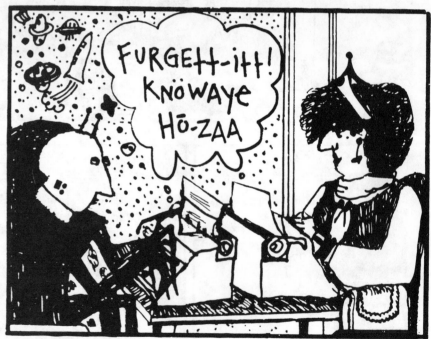

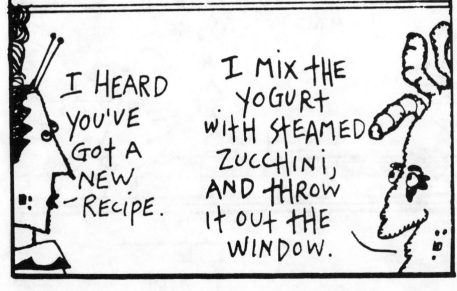

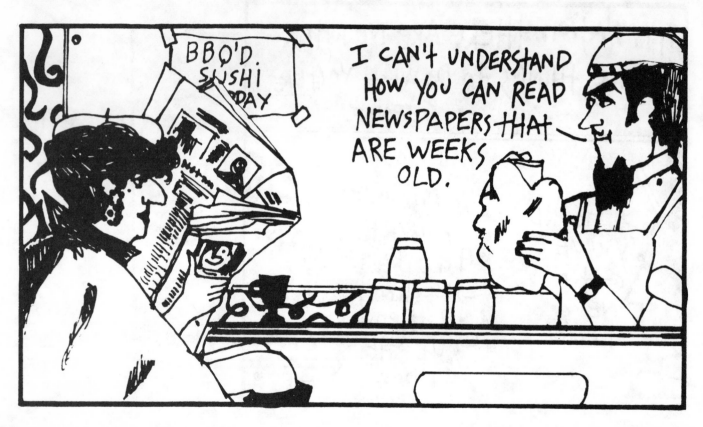

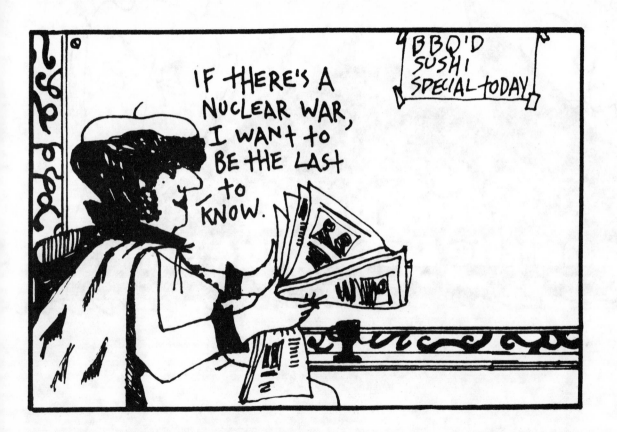

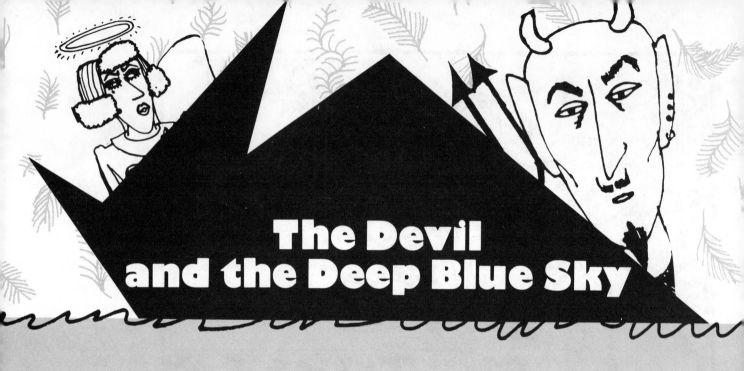

The Devil
and the Deep Blue Sky

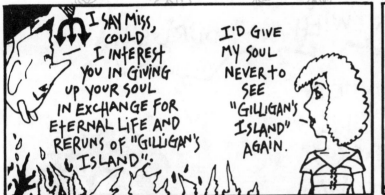

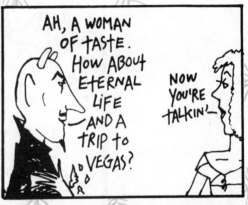

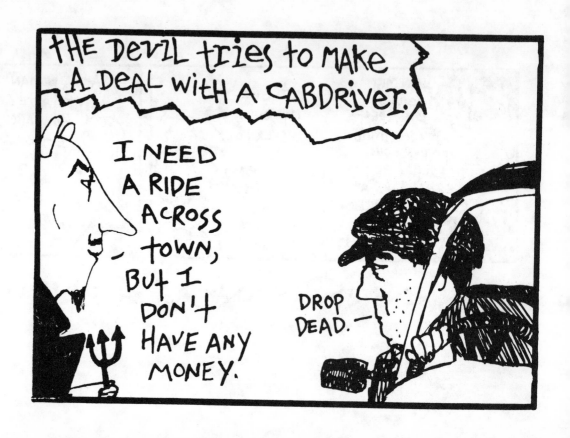

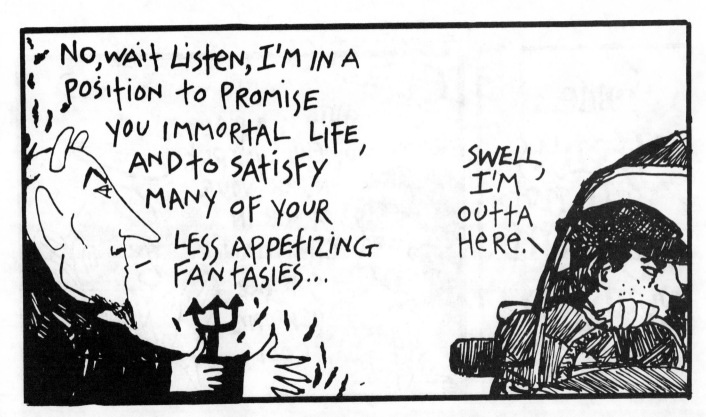

75

Some offenses will not go unpunished in Heaven

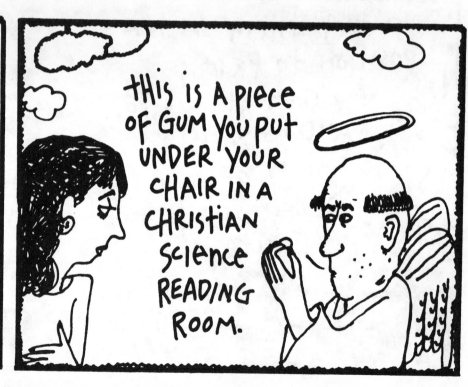

tHis is a piece of gum you put under your chair in a Christian Science Reading Room.

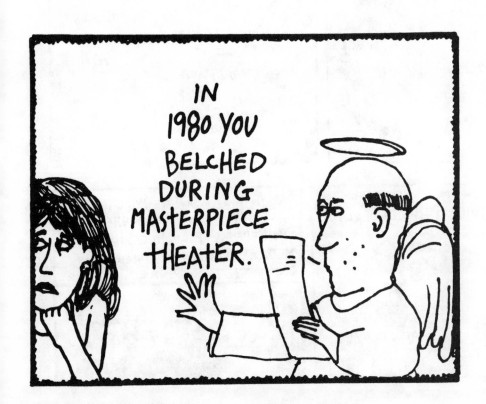

77

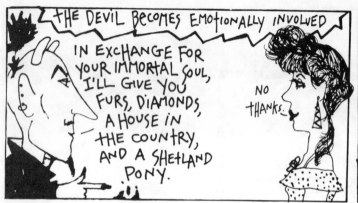

THE DEVIL BECOMES EMOTIONALLY INVOLVED

IN EXCHANGE FOR YOUR IMMORTAL SOUL, I'LL GIVE YOU FURS, DIAMONDS, A HOUSE IN THE COUNTRY, AND A SHETLAND PONY.

NO THANKS.

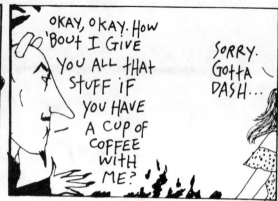

OKAY, OKAY. HOW 'BOUT I GIVE YOU ALL THAT STUFF IF YOU HAVE A CUP OF COFFEE WITH ME?

SORRY. GOTTA DASH...

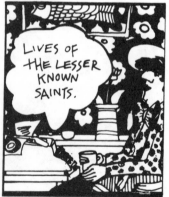

LIVES OF THE LESSER KNOWN SAINTS.

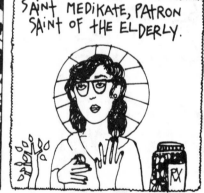

SAINT MEDIKATE, PATRON SAINT OF THE ELDERLY.

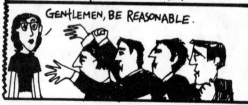

MARTYRED BY A SENATE SUB-COMMITTEE WHILE TRYING TO EXPLAIN THE SHORT-SIGHTEDNESS OF CUTTING PREVENTIVE MEDICAL SERVICES AND PRESCRIPTION DRUGS OUT OF MEDICARE.

GENTLEMEN, BE REASONABLE.

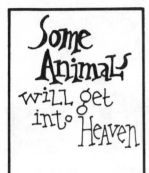

Some Animals will get into Heaven

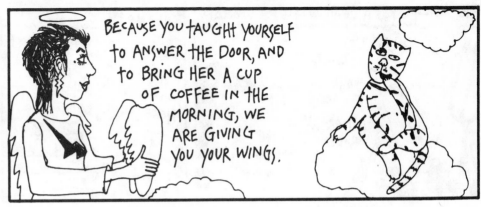

BECAUSE YOU TAUGHT YOURSELF TO ANSWER THE DOOR, AND TO BRING HER A CUP OF COFFEE IN THE MORNING, WE ARE GIVING YOU YOUR WINGS.

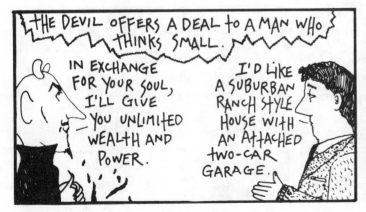

THE DEVIL OFFERS A DEAL TO A MAN WHO THINKS SMALL.

IN EXCHANGE FOR YOUR SOUL, I'LL GIVE YOU UNLIMITED WEALTH AND POWER.

I'D LIKE A SUBURBAN RANCH STYLE HOUSE WITH AN ATTACHED TWO-CAR GARAGE.

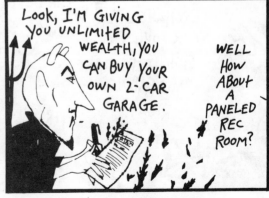

LOOK, I'M GIVING YOU UNLIMITED WEALTH, YOU CAN BUY YOUR OWN 2-CAR GARAGE.

WELL HOW ABOUT A PANELED REC ROOM?

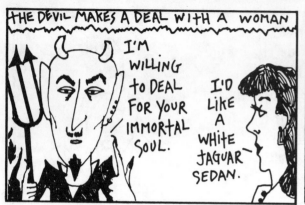
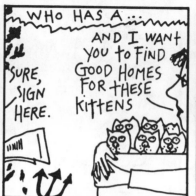
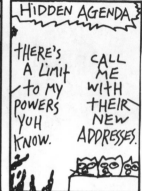
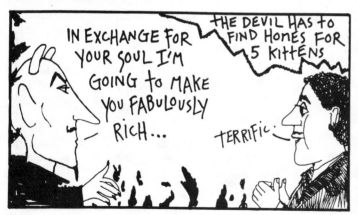
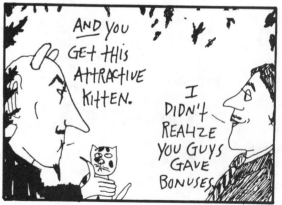

80

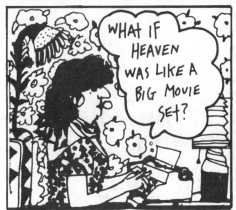

WHAT IF HEAVEN WAS LIKE A BIG MOVIE SET?

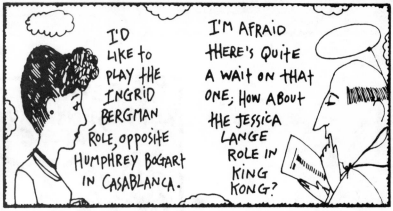

I'D LIKE TO PLAY THE INGRID BERGMAN ROLE, OPPOSITE HUMPHREY BOGART IN CASABLANCA.

I'M AFRAID THERE'S QUITE A WAIT ON THAT ONE; HOW ABOUT THE JESSICA LANGE ROLE IN KING KONG?

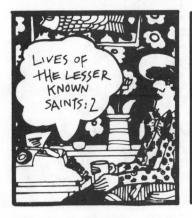

LIVES OF THE LESSER KNOWN SAINTS: 2

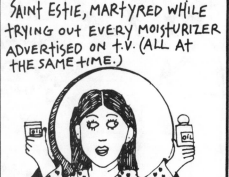

SAINT ESTIE, MARTYRED WHILE TRYING OUT EVERY MOISTURIZER ADVERTISED ON T.V. (ALL AT THE SAME TIME.)

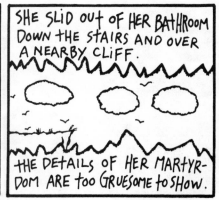

SHE SLID OUT OF HER BATHROOM DOWN THE STAIRS AND OVER A NEARBY CLIFF.

THE DETAILS OF HER MARTYRDOM ARE TOO GRUESOME TO SHOW.

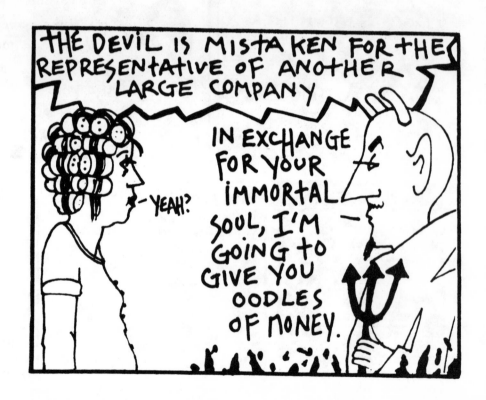

82

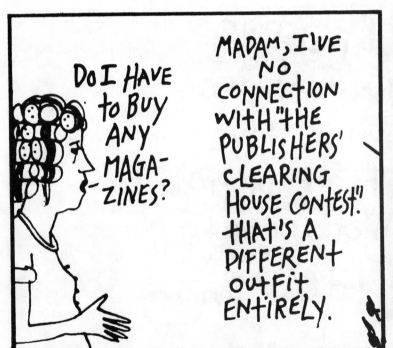

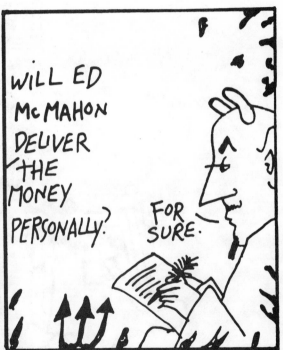

83

the MEMBERS
of Some
Institutions
wiLL HAve
Lots oF DiFFicuLty
getting iNto
Heaven

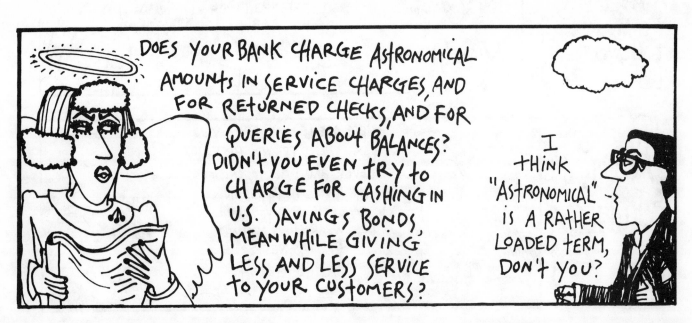

85

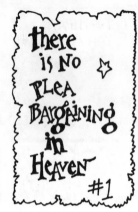

there is NO PLEA Bargaining in Heaven #1

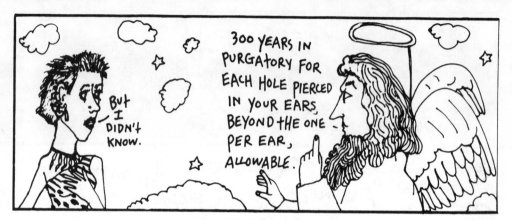

BUT I DIDN'T KNOW.

300 YEARS IN PURGATORY FOR EACH HOLE PIERCED IN YOUR EARS, BEYOND THE ONE PER EAR, ALLOWABLE.

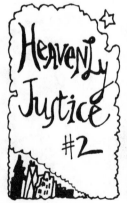

Heavenly Justice #2

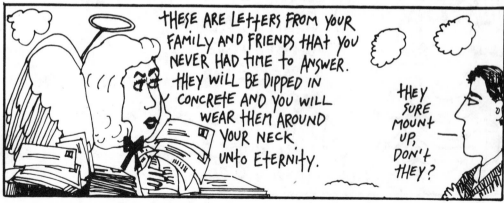

THESE ARE LETTERS FROM YOUR FAMILY AND FRIENDS THAT YOU NEVER HAD TIME TO ANSWER. THEY WILL BE DIPPED IN CONCRETE AND YOU WILL WEAR THEM AROUND YOUR NECK UNTO ETERNITY.

THEY SURE MOUNT UP, DON'T THEY?

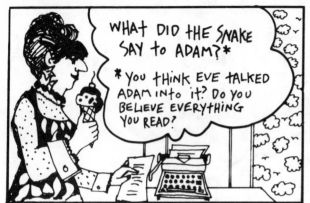

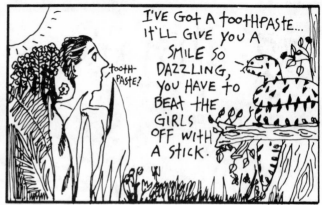

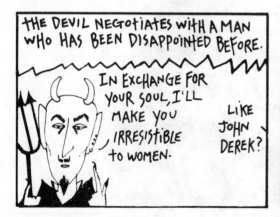

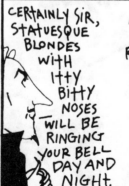

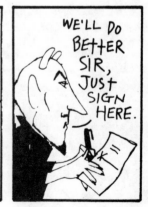

Big Mistakes in Biblical Times

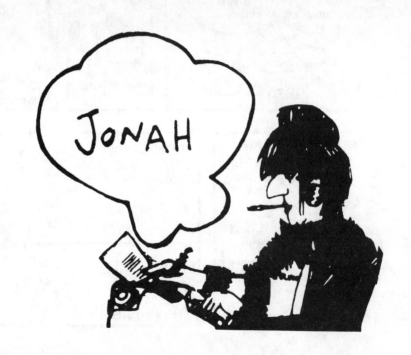

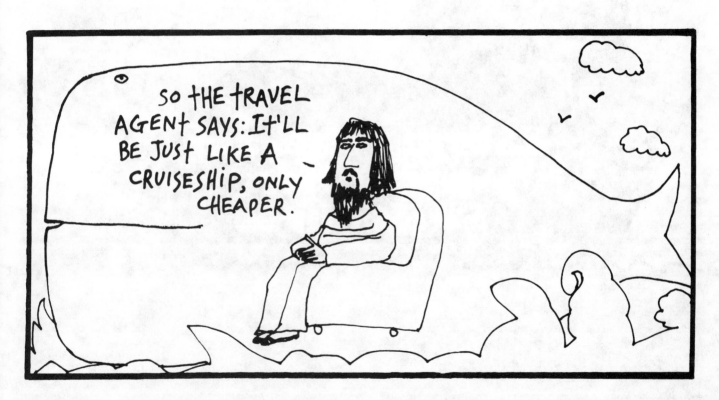

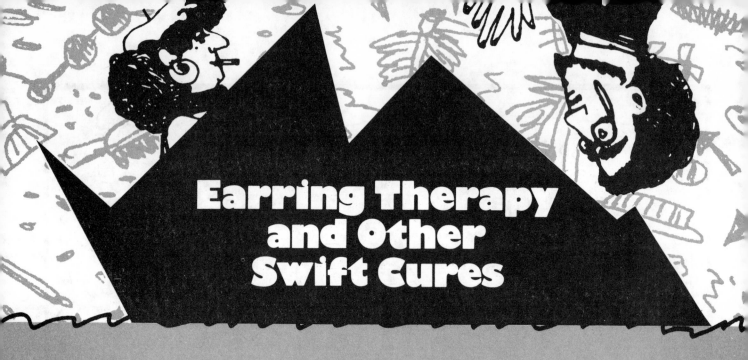

Earring Therapy and Other Swift Cures

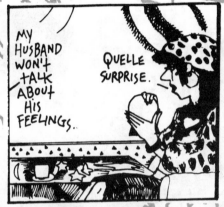

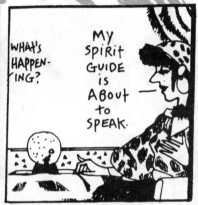

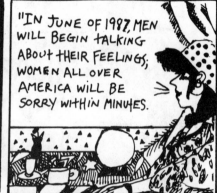

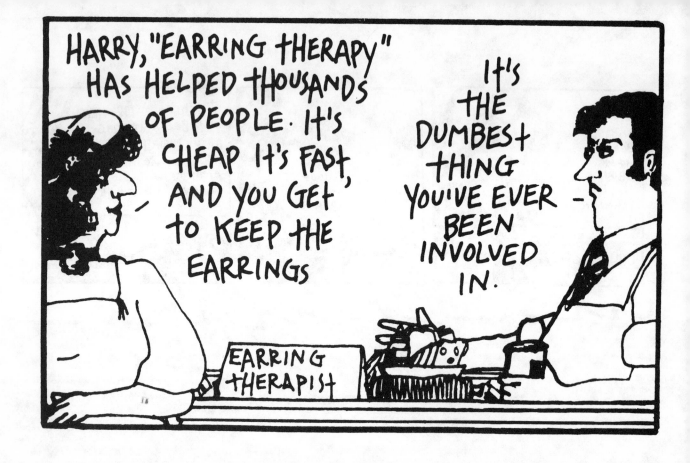

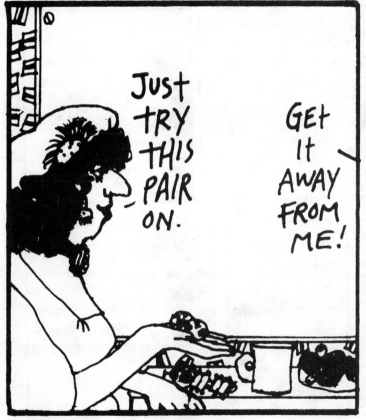

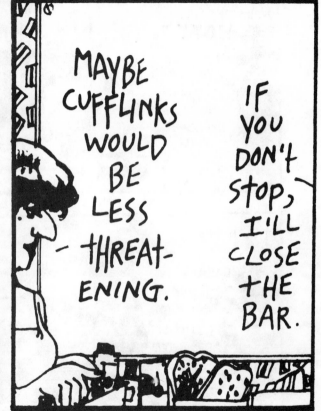

93

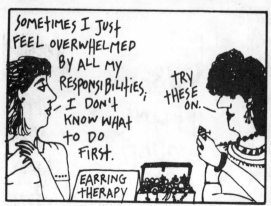

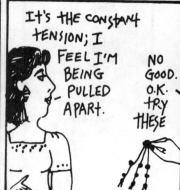

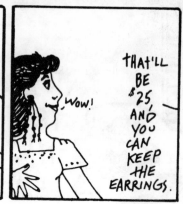

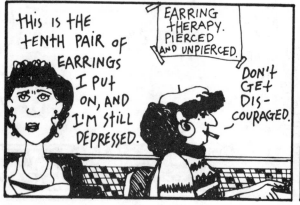

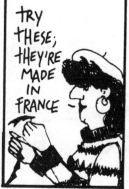

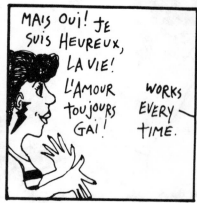

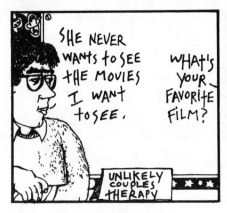

SHE NEVER WANTS TO SEE THE MOVIES I WANT TO SEE.

WHAT'S YOUR FAVORITE FILM?

UNLIKELY COUPLES THERAPY

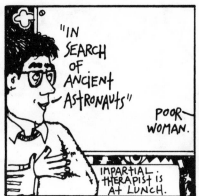

"IN SEARCH OF ANCIENT ASTRONAUTS"

POOR WOMAN.

IMPARTIAL THERAPIST IS AT LUNCH.

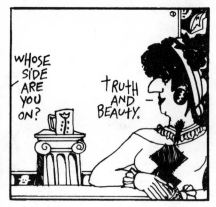

WHOSE SIDE ARE YOU ON?

TRUTH AND BEAUTY.

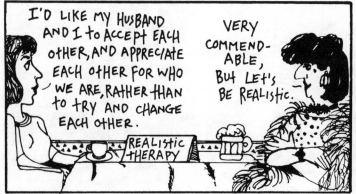

I'D LIKE MY HUSBAND AND I TO ACCEPT EACH OTHER, AND APPRECIATE EACH OTHER FOR WHO WE ARE, RATHER THAN TO TRY AND CHANGE EACH OTHER.

VERY COMMEND-ABLE, BUT LET'S BE REALISTIC.

REALISTIC THERAPY

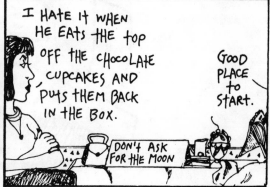

I HATE IT WHEN HE EATS THE TOP OFF THE CHOCOLATE CUPCAKES AND PUTS THEM BACK IN THE BOX.

GOOD PLACE TO START.

DON'T ASK FOR THE MOON

DREAMS OF FAMOUS PEOPLE

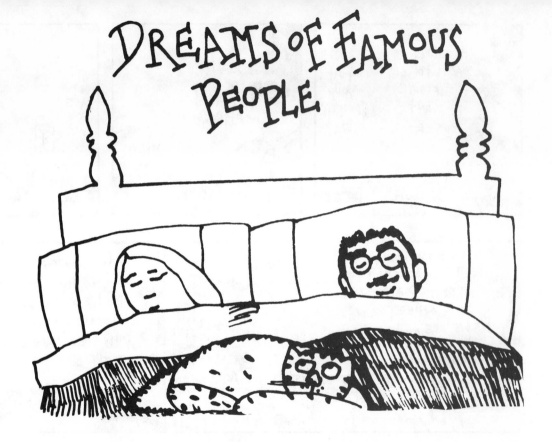

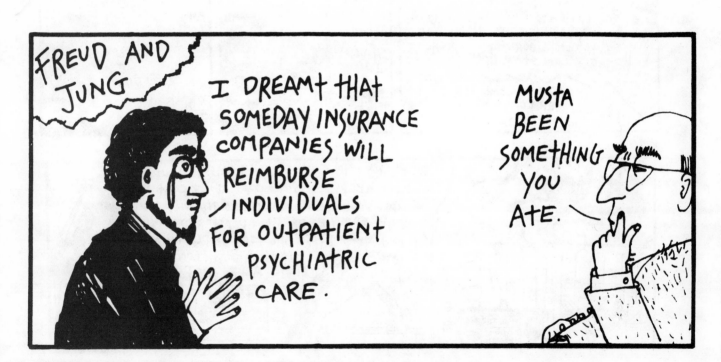

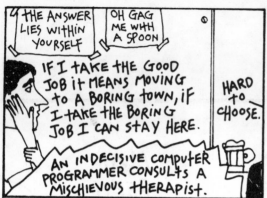

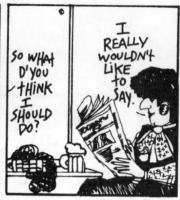

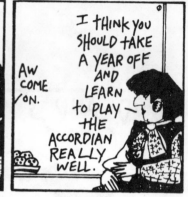

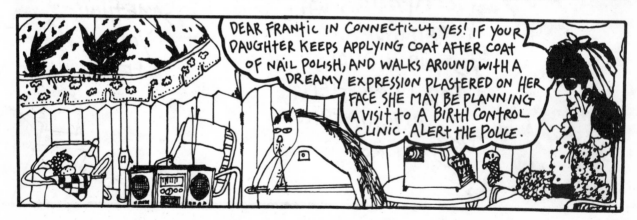

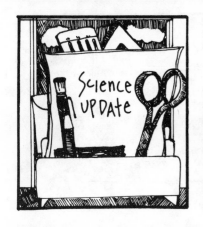

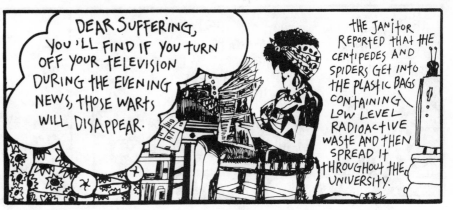

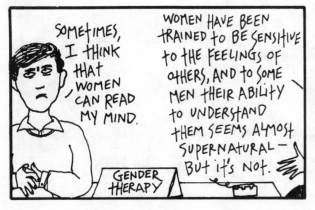

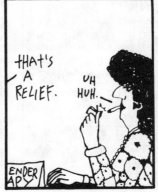

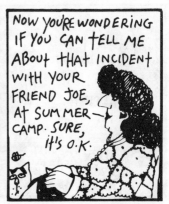

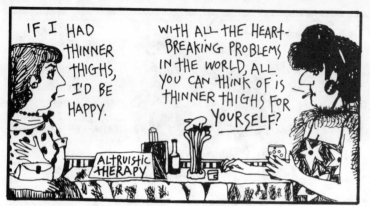

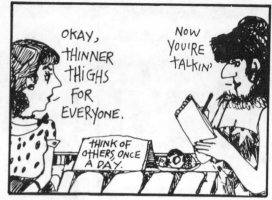

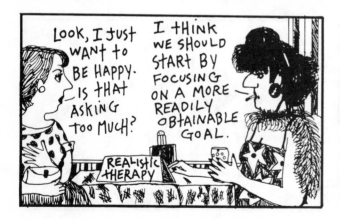

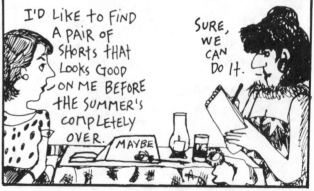

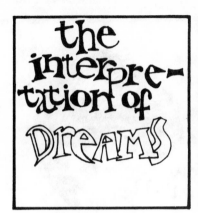

the inter-pre-tation of DReAMS

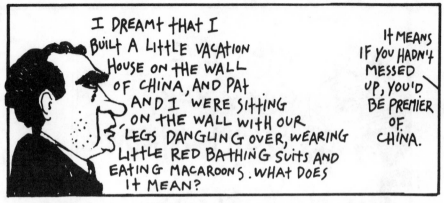

I DREAMt THAT I BUILt A LIttLE VACAtION HOUSE ON tHE WALL OF CHINA, AND PAt AND I WERE SItTING ON tHE WALL WItH OUR LEGS DANGLING OVER, WEARING LIttLE RED BAtHING SUItS AND EAtING MACAROONS. WHAt DOES It MEAN?

It MEANS IF YOU HADN't MESSED UP, YOU'D BE PREMIER OF CHINA.

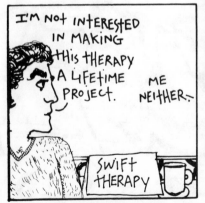

I'M NOt INtERESTED IN MAKING tHIS tHERAPY A LIFEtIME PROJECT.

ME NEItHER.

SWIFT THERAPY

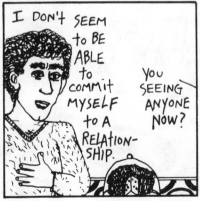

I DON't SEEM tO BE ABLE tO COMMIt MYSELF tO A RELAtION-SHIP.

YOU SEEING ANYONE NOW?

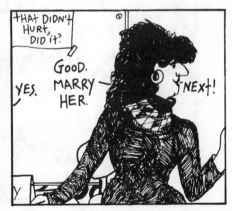

tHAt DIDN't HURT, DID It?

YES.

GOOD. MARRY HER.

NEXt!

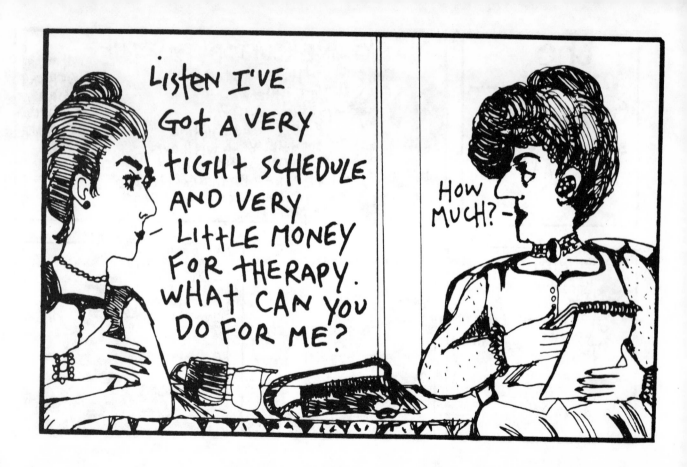

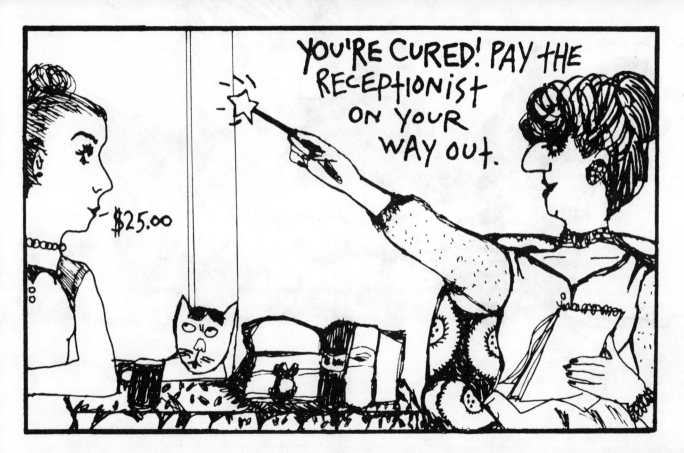

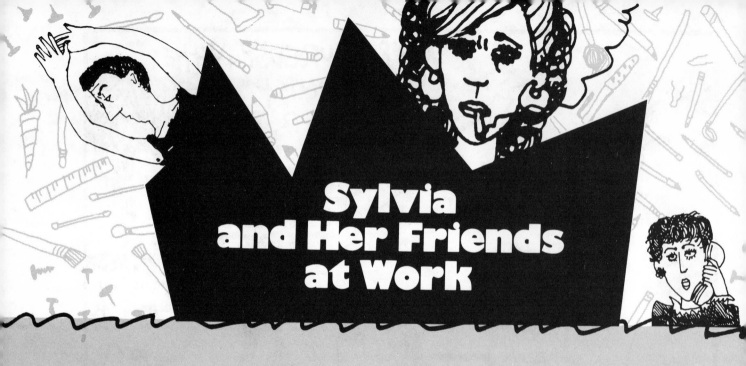

Sylvia
and Her Friends
at Work

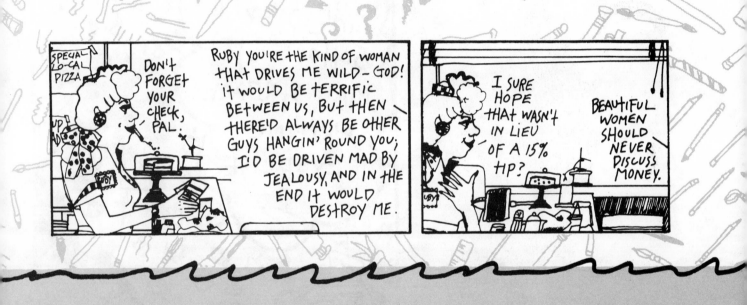

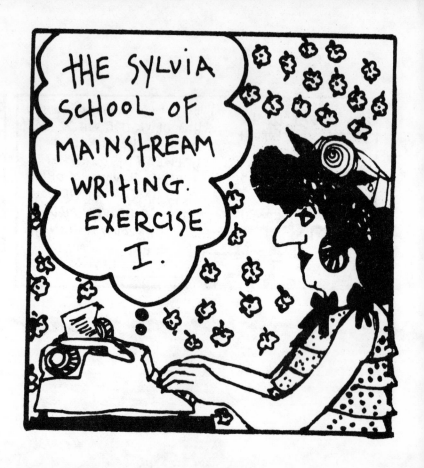

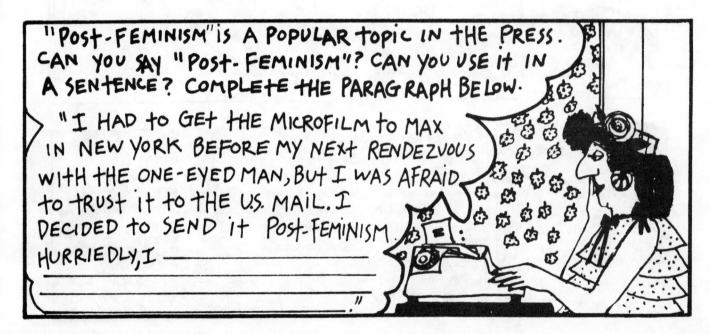

"POST-FEMINISM" IS A POPULAR topic IN THE PRESS. CAN YOU SAY "POST-FEMINISM"? CAN YOU USE IT IN A SENTENCE? COMPLETE THE PARAGRAPH BELOW.

"I HAD to GET THE MICROFILM to MAX IN NEW YORK BEFORE MY NEXT RENDEZVOUS WITH THE ONE-EYED MAN, BUT I WAS AFRAID to TRUST it to THE U.S. MAIL. I DECIDED to SEND it POST-FEMINISM. HURRIEDLY, I _____
_____
_____"

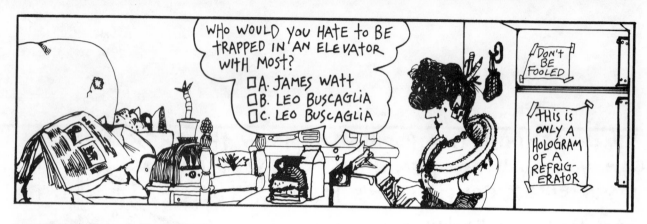

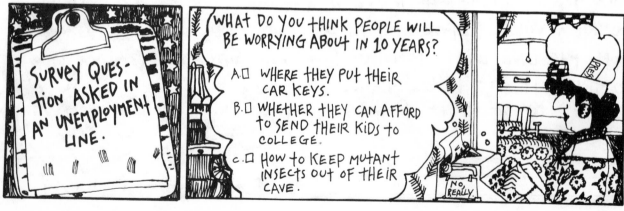

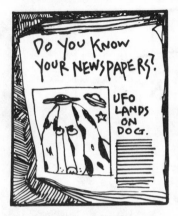

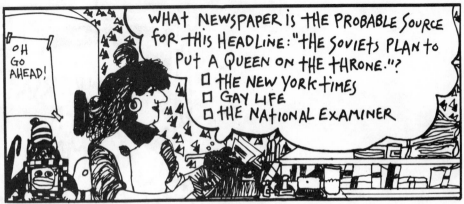

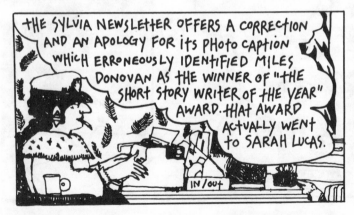

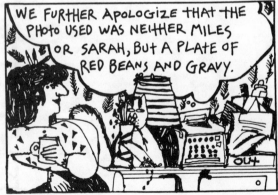

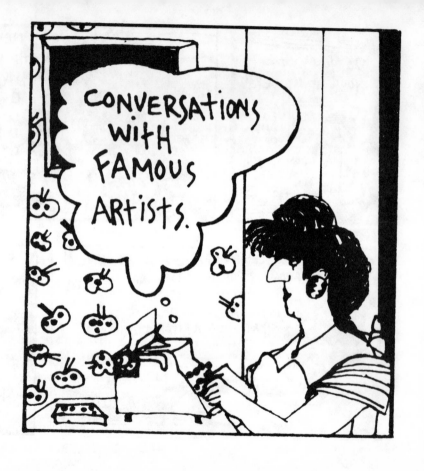

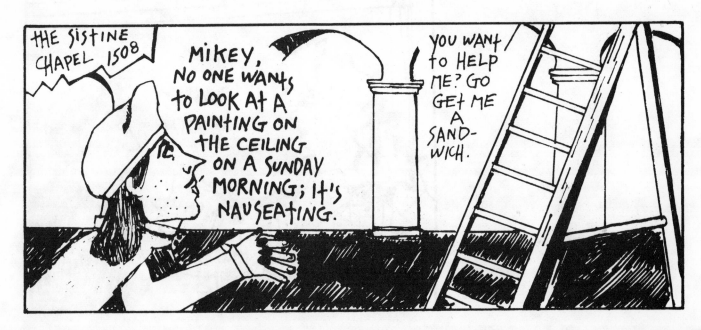

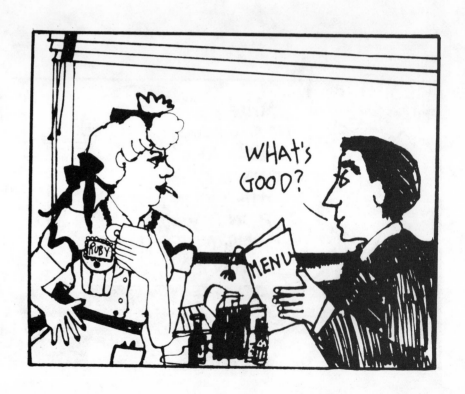

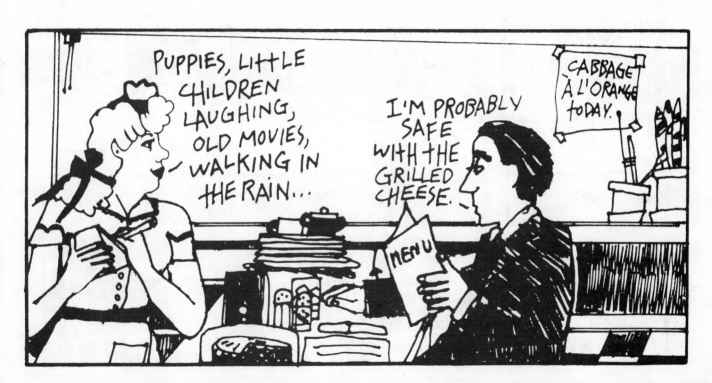

113

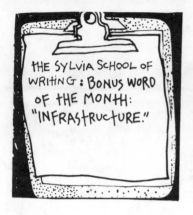

THE SYLVIA SCHOOL OF WRITING: BONUS WORD OF THE MONTH: "INFRASTRUCTURE."

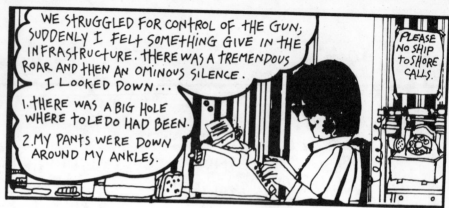

WE STRUGGLED FOR CONTROL OF THE GUN; SUDDENLY I FELT SOMETHING GIVE IN THE INFRASTRUCTURE. THERE WAS A TREMENDOUS ROAR AND THEN AN OMINOUS SILENCE. I LOOKED DOWN...

1. THERE WAS A BIG HOLE WHERE TOLEDO HAD BEEN.

2. MY PANTS WERE DOWN AROUND MY ANKLES.

PLEASE NO SHIP TO SHORE CALLS.

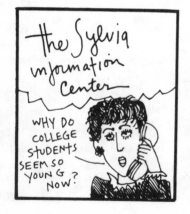

The Sylvia information Center

WHY DO COLLEGE STUDENTS SEEM SO YOUNG NOW?

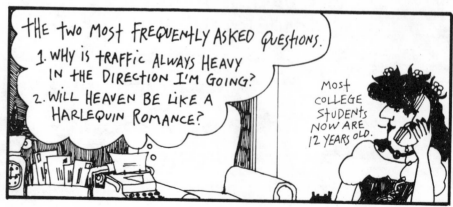

THE TWO MOST FREQUENTLY ASKED QUESTIONS.

1. WHY IS TRAFFIC ALWAYS HEAVY IN THE DIRECTION I'M GOING?

2. WILL HEAVEN BE LIKE A HARLEQUIN ROMANCE?

MOST COLLEGE STUDENTS NOW ARE 12 YEARS OLD.

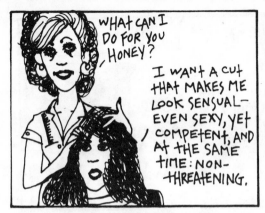

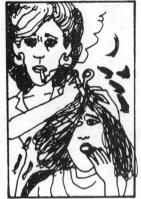

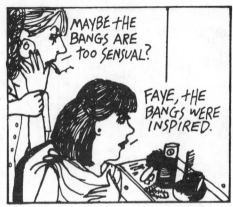

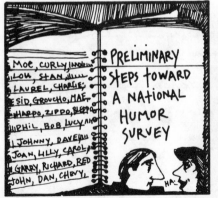

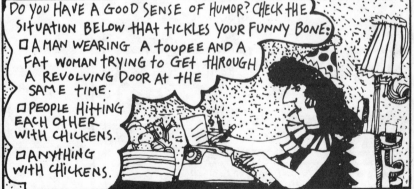

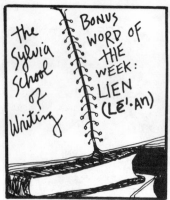

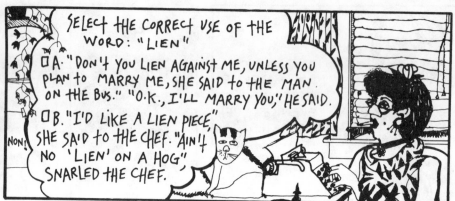

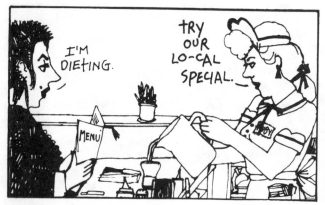

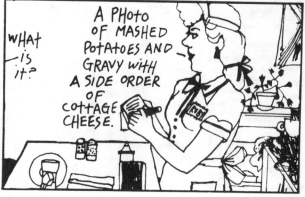

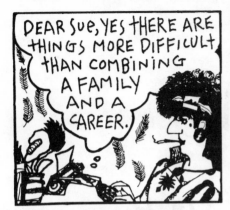

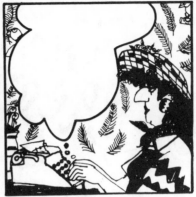

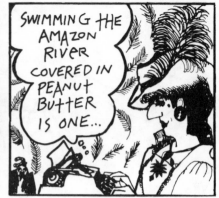

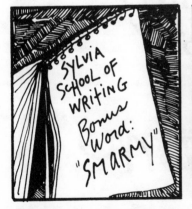

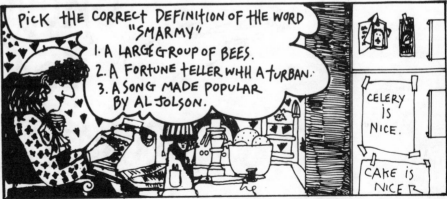

the Results of thought- less Positivism

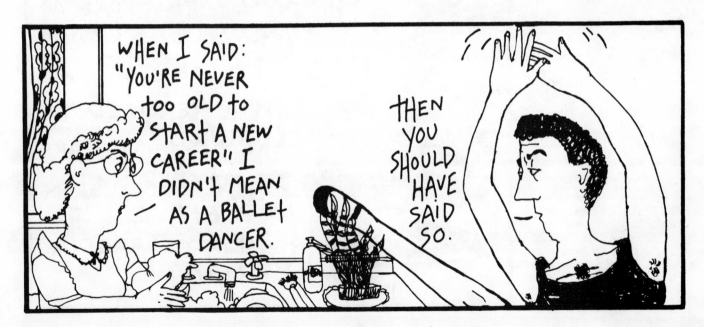

119

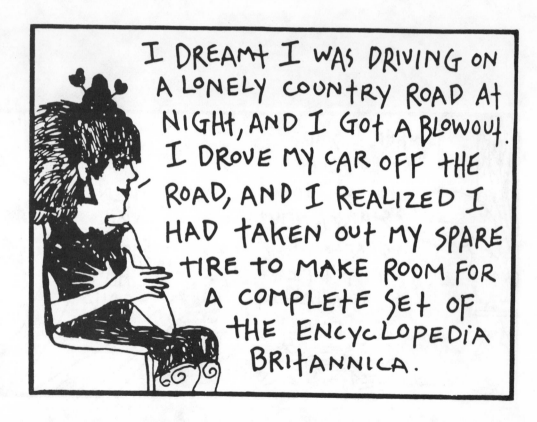

I DREAMT I WAS DRIVING ON A LONELY COUNTRY ROAD AT NIGHT, AND I GOT A BLOWOUT. I DROVE MY CAR OFF THE ROAD, AND I REALIZED I HAD TAKEN OUT MY SPARE TIRE TO MAKE ROOM FOR A COMPLETE SET OF THE ENCYCLOPEDIA BRITANNICA.

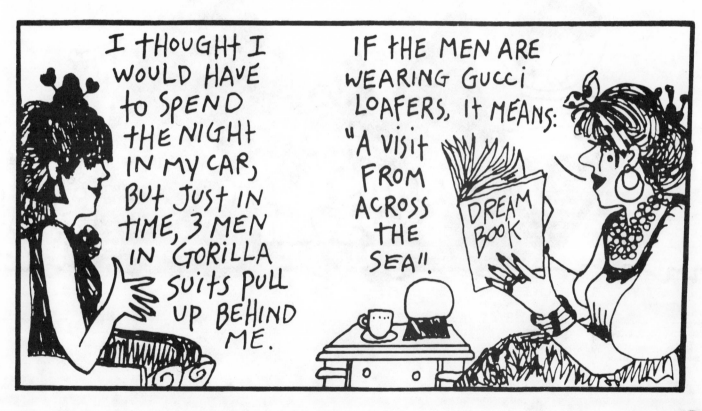

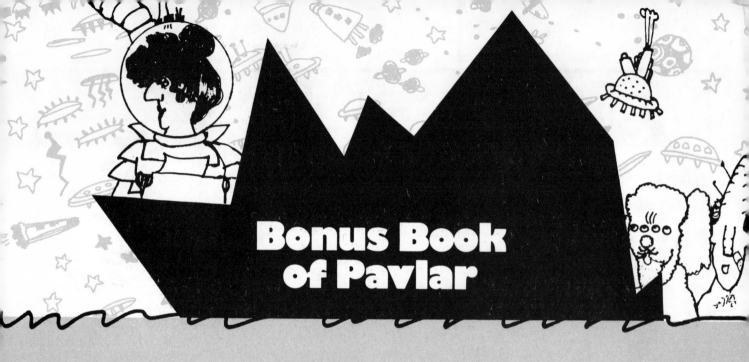

Bonus Book of Pavlar

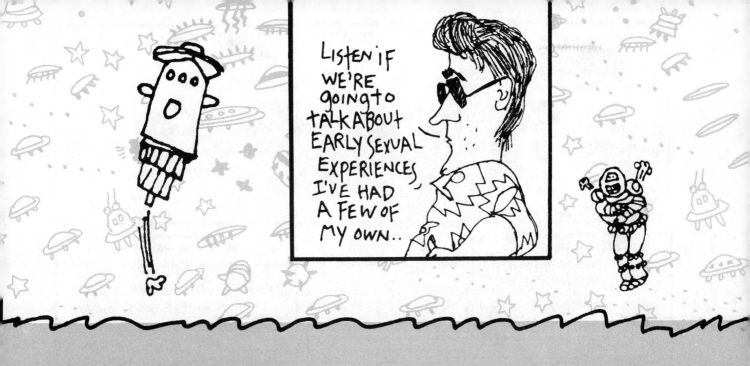

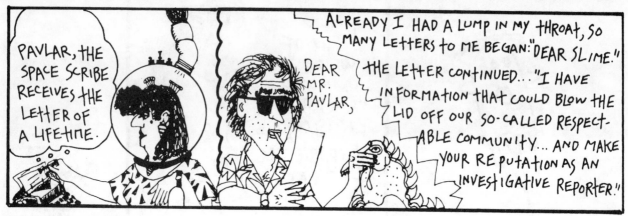

PAVLAR, THE SPACE SCRIBE RECEIVES THE LETTER OF A LIFETIME.

DEAR MR. PAVLAR,

ALREADY I HAD A LUMP IN MY THROAT, SO MANY LETTERS TO ME BEGAN: "DEAR SLIME." THE LETTER CONTINUED... "I HAVE INFORMATION THAT COULD BLOW THE LID OFF OUR SO-CALLED RESPECTABLE COMMUNITY... AND MAKE YOUR REPUTATION AS AN INVESTIGATIVE REPORTER."

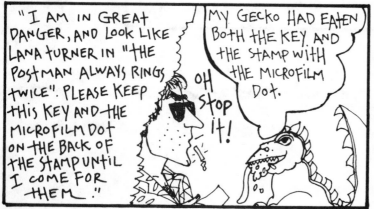

"I AM IN GREAT DANGER, AND LOOK LIKE LANA TURNER IN "THE POSTMAN ALWAYS RINGS TWICE". PLEASE KEEP THIS KEY AND THE MICROFILM DOT ON THE BACK OF THE STAMP UNTIL I COME FOR THEM."

OH STOP IT!

MY GECKO HAD EATEN BOTH THE KEY AND THE STAMP WITH THE MICROFILM DOT.

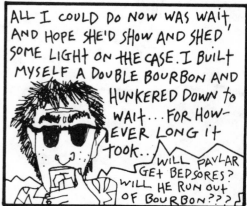

ALL I COULD DO NOW WAS WAIT, AND HOPE SHE'D SHOW AND SHED SOME LIGHT ON THE CASE. I BUILT MYSELF A DOUBLE BOURBON AND HUNKERED DOWN TO WAIT... FOR HOWEVER LONG IT TOOK..

WILL PAVLAR GET BEDSORES? WILL HE RUN OUT OF BOURBON???

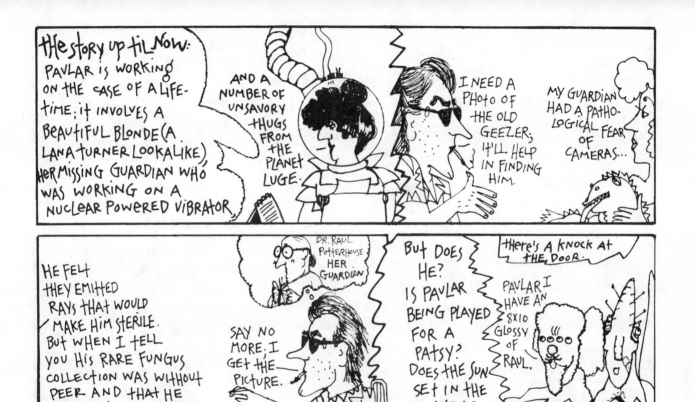

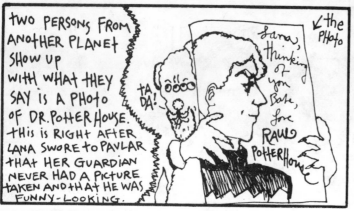

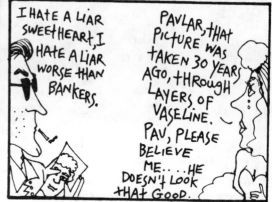

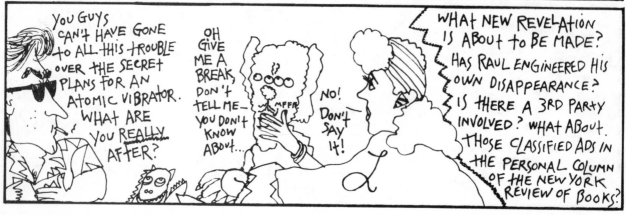

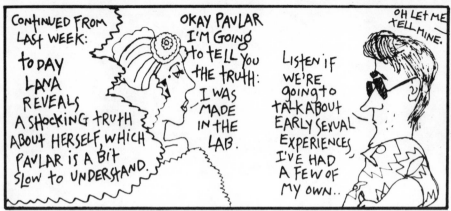
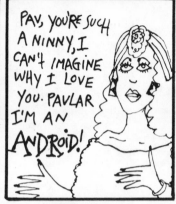

CONTINUED FROM LAST WEEK: TODAY LANA REVEALS A SHOCKING TRUTH ABOUT HERSELF, WHICH PAVLAR IS A BIT SLOW TO UNDERSTAND.

OKAY PAVLAR I'M GOING TO TELL YOU THE TRUTH: I WAS MADE IN THE LAB.

LISTEN IF WE'RE GOING TO TALK ABOUT EARLY SEXUAL EXPERIENCES, I'VE HAD A FEW OF MY OWN..

OH LET ME TELL MINE.

PAV, YOU'RE SUCH A NINNY, I CAN'T IMAGINE WHY I LOVE YOU. PAVLAR I'M AN ANDROID!

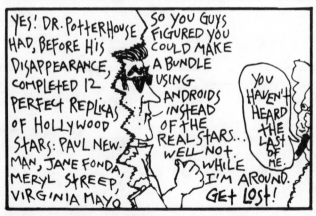
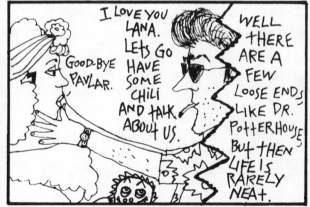

YES! DR. POTTERHOUSE HAD, BEFORE HIS DISAPPEARANCE, COMPLETED 12 PERFECT REPLICAS OF HOLLYWOOD STARS: PAUL NEWMAN, JANE FONDA, MERYL STREEP, VIRGINIA MAYO

SO YOU GUYS FIGURED YOU COULD MAKE A BUNDLE USING ANDROIDS INSTEAD OF THE REAL STARS... WELL NOT WHILE I'M AROUND. GET LOST!

YOU HAVEN'T HEARD THE LAST OF ME.

I LOVE YOU LANA. LETS GO HAVE SOME CHILI AND TALK ABOUT US.

GOOD-BYE PAVLAR.

WELL THERE ARE A FEW LOOSE ENDS, LIKE DR. POTTERHOUSE BUT THEN LIFE IS RARELY NEAT.